GET WITH THE
PROGRAM!

GETTING REAL ABOUT YOUR WEIGHT, HEALTH, AND EMOTIONAL WELL-BEING

BOB GREENE

SIMON & SCHUSTER

New York   London   Toronto   Sydney

This publication contains the opinions and ideas of its author. It is intended to provide helpful and informative material on the subjects addressed in the publication. It is sold with the understanding that the author and publisher are not engaged in rendering medical, health, psychological, or any other kind of personal professional services in the book. If the reader requires personal medical, health, or other assistance or advice, a competent professional should be consulted.

The author and publisher specifically disclaim all responsibility for any liability, loss, or risk, personal or otherwise, that is incurred as a consequence, directly or indirectly, of the use and application of any of the contents of this book.

SIMON & SCHUSTER
Rockefeller Center
1230 Avenue of the Americas
New York, NY 10020

Copyright © 2002 by Bob Greene
All rights reserved, including the right of reproduction in whole or in part in any form.

First Simon & Schuster trade paperback edition 2004

SIMON & SCHUSTER and colophon are registered trademarks
of Simon & Schuster, Inc.

MAKE THE CONNECTION and GET WITH THE PROGRAM
are registered trademarks of Harpo, Inc.

For information regarding special discounts for bulk purchases,
please contact Simon & Schuster Special Sales at
1-800-456-6798 or business@simonandschuster.com

Designed by Lisa Chovnick

Manufactured in the United States of America

10 9 8 7 6 5 4 3 2 1

The Library of Congress has cataloged the hardcover edition as follows:
Greene, Bob
Get with the program! : getting real about your weight, health, and
emotional well-being / Bob Greene.
221 p. : ill. ; 25 cm
Includes index.
1. Physical fitness. 2. Exercise. 3. Health I. Title
GV481 .G742   2002   613.7—dc21   2002283335
ISBN 0-7432-2599-6
      0-7432-3804-4 (Pbk)

ACKNOWLEDGMENTS

With special thanks to Maureen O'Brien, Chris Domingue, and the Santa Barbara Athletic Club for their contributions to this work. In addition, I would like to thank my clients who share their unique stories with me, and now you, and continue to be a source of inspiration in my life.

CONTENTS

INTRODUCTION

Congratulations! Whether you realize it or not, simply by picking up this book you have taken the first of what I hope will be many steps, both large and small, simple and challenging, toward the most rewarding journey of all—the road to reclaiming your physical health, well-being, and happiness.

Living the best life possible is everyone's dream, and that includes maintaining a healthy weight; getting in shape; achieving strength, fitness, and self-assurance; and attaining a sense of feeling a whole lot better in general. Those goals are exactly what *Get with the Program* is all about.

This is not a diet book.

This is not a fitness book.

This is a book about moving—in the right direction. It's a book about getting real about getting back in shape, physically and emotionally, realistically and gradually. It's also a wake-up call and a reminder about many things that you may have already learned over the years but have, for whatever reason, put on the back burner for a while or let slide. It's a book about tuning into and tuning up your body day by day and little by little, until, before you know it, your extra weight begins melting away. It's also a book about changing the way you think—not only to help you make intelligent, healthy choices about how best to nourish and strengthen your body and to nurture your sense of well-being and self-esteem, but how to help you literally *move out of your own way.*

For as you probably already know, the best reason in the world to move—perhaps the most difficult exercise of all—is to learn how to push away the emotional obstacles that have been holding you back from accomplishing your personal goals. We all struggle with that challenge, believe me. The ultimate goal of *Get with the Program* is to help you get real about the changes you want to make in your life—once and for all. Do that at your own pace but with complete commitment to this program, and I promise that you will soon become slimmer, stronger, and brimming with self-assurance.

When you get with the program, you will get in touch with your inner self. When you acknowledge and identify the emotional issues and triggers that have caused you to overeat when you are no longer physically hungry and begin losing weight through sensible eating and exercise, you will have achieved one of the greatest accomplishments of all. In doing so, the personal benefits and physical rewards that will follow will be lifelong and life changing. Emotional overeating is an epidemic in the United States, and simply acknowledging that it might also be an issue for you is a major milestone along your journey to renewed health and happiness.

So, once again, I want to congratulate you for taking your first step toward becoming the best that you can be: stronger, slimmer, healthier, and happier. One step at a time. Realistically. Gradually. Consciously. Finally.

If you're serious about losing weight and keeping it off for good, I'm going to show you exactly how to do it—and why to do it. I can assure you that you are capable of doing everything that I teach you and—best of all—you will happily be able to do it for the rest of your life. I'm not selling anything trendy or something that promises unbelievable results with little or no work. There are no gimmicks here. You're going to be challenged in many different ways; that's always the case when you make meaningful changes to your life. What I'm offering you is good, sound, honest advice. And should you decide to follow this advice, it will change your life!

Get with the Program is not a quick fix. Let's face it, you've probably tried the quick-fix approach to dieting and know it never really works for long. My philosophy with this program is more along the lines of "slow and steady wins the race." It's about putting one foot in the front of the other, at your own pace, in your own time frame.

This program may or may not get you down to your "dream" weight. But realize that dreams can be elusive and so can a size-eight dress or a thirty-two-inch waist. Shooting for unrealistic goals is how the dreaded "yo-yo dieting" syndrome begins, and I'm sure you're familiar with that losing game. What we're trying for here are achievable results, results that you can live with comfortably.

Get with the Program is not about trying to get you to be "thin as a pin." You will find as you read further that my main motives are these: Move a little, lose a little. (Great.) Move a little more, lose a little more. (Even better.) Eat less, weigh less. (Naturally.) Stress and worry less, binge less. (Wonderful.) Weigh less, move more. Move more, eat more (but sensibly). Strength train more, metabolize more (and age less). And on and on until you soon discover that you're smiling more and looking great and feeling better than you have in ages.

This is a program for life, for people of every weight, size, shape, and age. When you Get with the Program, you will follow a simple progression of behavioral, exercise, and eating changes that will guide you through the following goals.

The Goals

1. Get real about adjusting your thought patterns to help create positive change.
2. Get stronger and healthier.
3. Get in touch with your emotional eating triggers.
4. Get on with finally living and feeling really good about yourself.

Who wouldn't want to achieve all four of these goals? Unfortunately, many people focus on the goal they believe is the most important one to them, which is usually losing weight, and they typically select the *quickest* way to do it. This is where their problems begin. If you're like the majority of people on this planet who have tried to lose weight, you have gone down this road at least once or twice and maybe ten or twenty times— only to eventually fail. If that's the case, I say let's go back to the drawing board and rethink that quick-fix way of thinking about weight loss.

First of all, isn't your *real* goal to live the best possible life? And wouldn't the best possible life include being a healthy and maintainable weight, being in shape, being in touch with your emotions, and feeling better about yourself? These four goals are all interrelated, and the best overall way to achieve any one of them is to go about achieving all of them *simultaneously.*

Get with the Program will help you accomplish all of those goals. It may not be the fastest way, but it is by far the best way. Trust me on that. This program is a recipe for success. You will become healthier, slimmer, happier, and stronger—mentally and physically. Don't worry about the daunting goal of trying to quickly get down to your ideal or fighting weight. Toss that goal out the window *now* and replace it with striving to be simply trimmer and stronger.

This program is especially geared for people who have found it difficult over the years to maintain their shape, weight, and strength, and who have tried numerous diets only to succeed for a short time and then to fail. If you include yourself on that list, you are certainly not alone. In fact, you have a lot of company, and this book was written for you.

Get with the Program is comprised of four clear-cut phases, which correspond directly to the program's four goals. Each phase requires that you make specific investments in yourself, which will physically and emotionally prepare you to successfully move on to the program's next phase and goal.

Phase One is about preparation—mental and physical. You'll begin with simple changes to your body and, more importantly, to your mindset. You won't change what or how you eat. You won't even do any formal physical exercise. You will, however, perform several written exercises that will help you learn as much as you can about yourself and your attitudes about the process of change. These exercises will help you get in touch with your personal issues with regard to your health, happiness, and any potentially self-destructive habits.

Simply put, this is the time for you to learn the truth about your real attitudes toward changing your life. In doing so, you will learn plenty about the actual process of weight loss and the specific obstacles that have been in your way. You will also begin to move by gradually increasing your usual amount of physical activity to strengthen and prepare your body for regular (or increased) exercise in the next phase. You might start by stashing your remote control in the closet and getting off the couch every time you want to change the channel on your television set. Or you might decide to climb the stairs to your office on the sixth floor every morning and afternoon instead of taking the elevator. Whatever it is, you decide. Just stick with your decision. Be faithful to it and to your health.

I will also ask you to sign an actual contract with yourself, committing to Get with the Program. You'd be surprised how motivating putting your intentions in writing can be. Oh, and yes, you'll also drink plenty of water—lots and lots of water.

In Phase Two, you'll learn how to exercise properly and what aerobic exercise can do for you, especially to kick-start your metabolism. As you progress through this phase, you will actually begin to see weight loss results as your body's metabolism increases. This metabolic boost will eventually lead to dramatic changes in your body. This is the time when you'll begin to modify your eating and drinking behavior—especially if you currently drink alcoholic beverages, which you will begin to limit at this stage. You will also continue to drink plenty of water.

In Phase Three, you will continue to follow and benefit from what you've already accomplished in the first two phases, as you begin to focus on the emotional connection to your eating habits and how they affect your overall health and fitness. In this part of the program, you will identify the emotional issues that trigger you to eat when you're not hungry—stress, anxiety, depression, boredom, loneliness, and fear of failure (or success!) are among the possibilities. By identifying and acknowledging those emotional trigger-points rather than by numbing yourself to them through snacking, overeating, and inactivity, you will soon find yourself making much better eating choices and decisions about how to treat your body. As you become physically and emotionally stronger and healthier, you will be better equipped to make a total commitment to fully impose your will to bring about permanent positive change to your life.

Finally, in Phase Four, you will continue to increase the amount of exercise that you perform, including the addition of strength training exercise. This is one of the program's keys to maintaining your weight loss success on a permanent basis, because it keeps your body's internal "metabolic fire" burning calories at a high level even when you're not exercising. This final phase will also find you focusing on fine-tuning your eating. The end result? A lifetime of health, well-being, strength, and stamina.

The four phases of the program remind me of the process of building a fire. Phase One is all about getting your inner fire going. It's when you strike that first match and spark the first flames. That flash of light that ignites the whole process. Phase Two is where you begin to fan and build up the fire, turning up the heat by adding fuel and oxygen to the flames. It's where you really get moving aerobically and start to stoke your inner furnace. Phase Three is where things really begin to burn in earnest as sparks start to fly and dance and the flames grow both in temperature and intensity. This is the stage where you get in touch with your hot buttons—where you discover why "emotional eating" has been weighing you down and what's really been "eating at" you. Finally, in Phase Four, your fire is ready for the really big logs—strength training exercises—which not only will help to make the fire burn brighter and stronger than it ever has done before, but will help to maintain the radiating glow and brilliant burn long after you have lifted those heavy logs and heaved them onto the fire.

Get with the Program is designed to get you where you want to go. It's a program that is designed to help you finally become the person you were always meant to be.

Now let's fire it up . . . and get going!

TRUTH, COMMITMENT, AND SELF-CONTROL

Phase One is about changing the way you think. It's about moving toward your goal of enjoying a healthier and happier future, by stretching and flexing your emotional muscles as well as increasing your physical activity.

You will begin this phase not by diving into a strict diet or a major workout program, but by embarking on a bit of soul-searching and self-discovery. Before you can learn the truth about how to lose weight and keep it off, you must first get in touch with some truths about yourself, and that will include making a lifelong commitment to taking better care of yourself by signing a contract with yourself. Get with the Program, as you will see, is an interactive program in which you will chronicle your thoughts, goals, issues, and obstacles, as well as document your progress along your journey to lifelong health and well-being through increased physical fitness and realistic weight loss.

In addition, you are going to start moving more—whether it's taking a fifteen-minute walk after dinner, taking the stairs to your office instead of the elevator, or even washing the car yourself. I will also ask you to think about your choices about the food and drink that you put into your body, and I will have you drinking more fresh water than you have probably been accustomed to. But most of all, Phase One will have you focusing on getting your *mind* moving in the right direction.

Creating positive behavior in your life is what makes the difference between a successful fitness and weight loss plan and a failed one. A common mistake people make is to attempt to change all their negative behaviors too quickly. This is one reason you won't change the way you eat right away. In addition, if you cut your calories without first increasing your amount of exercise, your metabolism begins to shut down. This is a common mistake that many people make when they start a new weight loss program. You need to boost your metabolism with exercise *before* you cut down on the amount of calories that you eat.

In fact, some people who follow *Get with the Program* may *never* need to cut back on their eating, while others may actually need to eat *more* once they get moving. Remember, this is about getting healthy and instilling positive behavior in your life with regard to your body and overall well-being.

It takes patience and time to lose weight the right way, and it is necessary to lose weight progressively, in phases. You didn't gain your extra weight overnight, so don't expect positive results to happen immediately.

You see, your body needs time to adjust to each new change that you make. Our bodies have evolved this way so that we can correctly interpret how to respond to environmental stresses that we may encounter. For example, let's say you want to lose weight and you decide to start by cutting calories. You would expect that limiting your food consumption would naturally result in weight loss. But the message that your body receives is that there is a food shortage, and it responds by protecting against the loss of body fat. It does so by shutting down the burning of calories. This is exactly what you *don't* want to happen. Thousands of years ago this may have been a valuable mechanism to protect against starvation, but now it presents a potential problem.

Since you don't want your body to go into starvation mode—conserving instead of burning fat—you should never start a weight loss program by cutting calories. Instead, you should begin by maintaining the calories that your body is accustomed to and adding more physical movement into your daily lifestyle—the more aerobic and challenging the exercise, the better. This tells your body that adequate food is available and that it should not slow down your metabolism. In fact, this is one of the basic foundations of Get with the Program. By increasing your daily physical activity—even in small ways—without starving yourself, you actually kick-start your metabolism. Gradually, you will find that the more your activity increases, the more your metabolism increases, and you will eventually experience *real* weight loss—or, more accurately, *fat* loss.

Later on in Phase Four, you will add weight training to your fitness regimen. But strength training usually increases your appetite, and I want your ability to make food choices to be really under control by the time you add that challenge. At that point, when you cut back a little on the amount of food that you do consume, the weight loss results will be dramatic and sustainable.

Get with the Program is all about patience, persistence and pacing. It's about self-discipline, self-control, and personal commitment. Most of all, it's about feeling good about yourself and taking good care of yourself. This program is a realistic life-changing process—for life!

Goals for Phase One

- Explore your beliefs, attitudes, and behaviors that relate to yourself and the process of change.
- Learn all about the process of how you gain and lose weight.
- Make a personal pledge to Get with the Program by signing a contract with yourself.
- Start drinking a minimum of 6 eight-ounce glasses of water each day.
- Start to improve your functional fitness by moving more and performing some basic exercises.
- Prepare yourself for a lifetime of being healthy and fit.

MOVE A LITTLE

Be it a little or a lot, the key ingredient to beginning the program is to get moving—and the more the better. At the end of this section, I will give you some specific instructions for a few basic moves that will help you to stretch and strengthen your body. In the meantime, from this day on, I want you to make a conscious decision to increase your physical activity as much as possible. Shoot for at least thirty minutes (broken into ten- or fifteen-minute segments if necessary) per day for now. The goal is to get yourself back on track, so just get up and move! For instance:

Hide your remote controls.

Walk instead of drive.

Take stairs instead of elevators.

Ride a bike.

Row a boat.

Jump rope.

Pull some weeds.

Polish a floor.

Paint a wall.

Wash a car.

Jog in place.

Splash around in a fountain.

Take a hike.

You get the picture. Just by exerting a little more energy every single day, you'll boost your metabolism. By moving more, you're getting with the program physically. Now it's time to start getting in step with the program mentally and emotionally.

ACQUIRING A HEALTHY ATTITUDE TOWARD YOURSELF AND THE PROCESS OF CHANGE

Have you ever started a diet or a fitness program and then failed to "stick with it"? Do you remember if your level of motivation was the strongest just before you started, slightly less when you actually began, and then nonexistent once the novelty wore off? This happens to a lot of people, and if it's ever happened to you, there's a good chance that your mental and emotional framework going into it was all wrong, as it is for the majority of people who attempt to lose weight. The bottom line is, if you want results and you want them to last, you'll probably need to first change the way you think.

In my twenty-plus years of helping people to lose weight, I've learned something very important. *The way that you think will ultimately dictate your long-term success or failure.* When I first begin to work with any new client, I spend up to two hours just gathering information about her. I look for what I call potential land mines. Just about everyone has at least one of these issues. These land mines are really attitudes, traits, beliefs, or behaviors that will eventually surface and sabotage their health and fitness goals in some way. The result can range from minor motivational setbacks to a complete abandonment of their goals. This is why we're going to deal with these issues now, before you invest the time, energy, and emotional commitment necessary to change your life. I want you to start by taking a little quiz designed to help you recognize any issues that negatively affect you and your potential for change.

Simply answer yes or no to each of the twelve questions below. Each question corresponds to a specific attitude, trait, belief, or behavior that may affect your level of motivation to move forward. After you take this quiz, read the section that follows in which I address the meaning of your answers to the questions, and then you can decide if further work is needed on your part. As you read the explanatory information about each question, look for anything that specifically applies to you. You may even find recurring themes in the way you answer or react to many of these questions. That's what this part of the program is designed to do, to get you thinking and to make sure that all your emotional ducks are in a row.

Circle Your Answer

1. Do you believe that once you reach a certain size or weight you'll be happy? **Yes No**

2. Do you frequently look for a shortcut or an easier way to achieve what you want? **Yes No**

3. Do you frequently use excuses to get yourself out of doing what it takes to reach your goals? **Yes No**

4. Are you often impatient with slow results? **Yes No**

5. Do you ever consider giving up when you experience minor setbacks? **Yes No**

6. Do you often procrastinate? **Yes No**

7. Are you afraid of change? **Yes No**

8. Do you typically choose immediate gratification over reaching your long-term goals? **Yes No**

9. Do you ever use family, relationship, or work obligations as an excuse not to take care of yourself? **Yes No**

10. Are you afraid of disappointing others? **Yes No**

11. Do you ever blame something or someone else for
    your inability to reach your goals? **Yes No**

12. Do you ever feel that you don't deserve to be
    happy or successful? **Yes No**

The preceding twelve questions were designed to identify potential attitudes, traits, and behaviors that can hold you back from achieving health and well-being. Many of these issues take time and effort to change. Recognizing the ones that need to change for you is the first step, but successfully changing behaviors and core beliefs requires desire, daily effort, patience, and perseverance. Plan the best course of action for addressing these issues and combine it with an aggressive program of caring for yourself. If you answered yes to any of the twelve questions, be sure to do the written exercise that corresponds to that question, preferably prior to moving on to Phase Two.

Each time you answered yes to one of the above questions, you've raised a little red flag. It may signal that your mind-set may not be optimal for long-term weight loss success or that you have unrealistic expectations about what that success entails. Most people are affected by at least one or more of these issues, so if you are, don't feel like you're alone. What you're trying to accomplish now is to recognize the issues that negatively affect you and that will need future work and attention on your part. Read the following section carefully and fully. Take the time to do the written exercise at the end of each section. It is designed to help initiate the process of changing your attitude. The time to start addressing your issues is now. And while in an ideal world you would have all these issues resolved by the end of Phase One, the truth is that change is a process. What you need to do before entering Phase Two of the program is at least understand the general concept behind each of the twelve questions presented here. As you progress through the program, you may find that you need to continue to pay attention to your emotional issues and well-being well into Phase Four, and that's fine. That's exactly what the program is all about—gradual progress toward positive change.

1. Do you believe that once you reach a certain size or weight, you'll be happy?

I can't tell you how often my clients either hint at or say outright that they'll be happy once they lose a specific amount of weight. As soon as I hear those words, a big red flag goes up in my mind. When you say to yourself, "I'll be happy when I reach _____ pounds," one of two outcomes can occur. The first is that you never reach that weight and are, therefore, never happy. The second outcome is that you reach that magical weight and realize after a while that it has absolutely nothing to do with your happiness. Eventually you slide back into your old habits and quickly put back on all the weight that you lost . . . and often then some. Either way, it's a no-win situation.

What I want you to fully understand is that your excess weight is usually a symptom of something else. If you address only the symptom (your excess weight), you'll never permanently solve anything. However, if you identify and deal with the underlying issue or problem, you'll not only be a happier individual, you'll be much more likely to care for yourself in such a way that your weight will no longer be such a struggle.

Keep in mind that the underlying issue (or issues) can be easy or difficult to resolve. You simply may have too much stress in your life or lack the willpower to turn down your favorite junk food. Be aware, however, that I have had many clients who believed that they simply lacked the proper discipline to turn down their favorite foods, when the truth was their dilemma was much more complex (such as that something—or someone—meaningful was missing from their life). They just never took the time and energy to explore their feelings, or they buried those feelings with food. Quite often part of what's missing is a healthy level of self-esteem, which also contributes to emotional eating (I'll talk more about emotional eating in Phase Three).

Whatever your excess weight is symptomatic of, it is important to get to the bottom of the reason and to determine what in your life needs to change. First, be willing to accept that your excess weight may be an emotional bandage of sorts to cover up an underlying issue. Next, work hard to identify what that issue might be. This is where the self-discovery process begins and continues . . . forever! That's right. Self-discovery doesn't end when you reach a certain weight or size, it is a lifetime pursuit. Finally, you need to make the commitment to change those things that negatively affect you, no matter how long it takes. Woven into this journey of self-discovery is a committment to exercising and eating healthy foods.

You need to recognize and to feel good about all of your accomplishments. It is also essential that you don't make your weight loss more important than it really is. Remember that it is only one way to feel good about yourself—you can create others. Otherwise, your emotions and feeling of self-worth will simply go up and down inversely with your weight, and the scale will become the source of your highs and lows. This is an emotional roller coaster you can't afford to take.

Be patient. If you can find or create things to be happy about today, you'll be much more likely to take care of yourself tomorrow.

I can't stress enough how important it is for you to establish a variety of goals in several aspects of your life. This will give you many more opportunities to feel good about yourself each day and will help take the pressure off your weight loss program. Take night classes, learn to play an instrument, join a social group, do that thing that you've always said you wanted to do. During this time it will be helpful to have a list of as many things as possible that make you feel good about yourself. This gives you that many more options to feel good each day. When you reach a road-block on one avenue, such as your weight loss program, you have other ways to get you down that self-esteem road. Enjoy the journey and you'll most certainly enjoy the destination.

WRITTEN EXERCISE

Make a list of all of the things you could do that would make you happy and that you feel would benefit your life. Include, in particular, those things that you've always said you wanted to do. Circle one or two of these and take the necessary steps to incorporate them into your life—*now.* Commit to a start date for each objective, then write down exactly what you need to do in order to put this goal in your life and hold yourself to it. Just be sure that one of the spaces includes to "Get with the Program"— and clear your schedule now!

Goal _____ **Start date** _____

What needs to be done _____

_____

_____

_____

Goal _____ Start date _____

What needs to be done _____

_____

_____

_____

Goal _____ Start date _____

What needs to be done _____

_____

_____

_____

Goal _____ Start date _____

What needs to be done _____

_____

_____

_____

2. Do you frequently look for a shortcut or an easier way to achieve what you want?

Dedication, commitment, and effort are needed to accomplish anything worthwhile. You need to work hard if you want to achieve success when it comes to raising your family and succeeding in your career. The same goes for maintaining a successful, loving relationship. Hard work is required to accomplish most anything worthwhile. Losing weight and taking care of yourself is no exception.

Memorize these words:

There are no shortcuts.

If you've ever tried any diet or weight loss fads, you're guilty of looking for a shortcut. Of course we've all, at one time or another, tried the latest diet, the newest pill, the hottest new fitness gadget, to little if any avail. Some people, though, are constantly searching for the easy way out. They simply jump from one gimmick to the next. They even go *back* to the same things that failed them the first time around! If your behavior at all resembles what I'm describing, listen up. When you are counting on your health, fitness, and weight loss goals to be accomplished by the latest fad, you are really looking for something to take the place of hard work and difficult choices. In other words, you don't have faith in yourself and in your own abilities. The easy way out will always look tempting when stacked up against hard work. But working hard and earning your results is *exactly* what increases your self-esteem. That sense of accomplishment is what will drive your results—not a shortcut.

Dale's Story

I had been working with Janice for about a year when she asked me if I could help her husband, Dale,* with his weight loss goals. I told her I could meet with him the next week. At that time, we would have a consultation and decide what the best course of action for him would be. I rarely commit to working with anyone before I've had the chance to meet with them and see if they are ready for the challenge of getting in shape and losing weight. When I met with Dale, he expressed a desire to lose forty pounds. He had gained this weight since he finished his law degree and started working at his father's law firm. During the consultation, I told Dale what he would need to do in order to make exercise part of his life and to reach his weight loss goals. Each time I would suggest a way to fit the exercise into his busy schedule, he would have a work-related objection as to why this was just not possible. His arguments always revolved around not having enough time. While I understood that he was busy, I felt that he simply could not commit to any plan that would result in his weight loss success. He asked me if I could work with him for half an hour, once a week, with the understanding that if something came up he would call and be able to cancel. I told him that wouldn't work for

---

* For privacy purposes, all names have been changed.

me and, even more important, it wouldn't work for *him*. We left without a commitment to begin exercising together.

I saw Dale from time to time over the course of the next year because we belonged to the same health club. Janice would tell me about Dale's latest diet or weight loss plan; I can remember at least six of them over the course of one year, each one ending with Dale's frustration and his gaining back any weight that he lost, and then some. I had also seen Dale with three other personal trainers that same year. It was obvious to me, and to Janice, that Dale avoided the hard work of changing either his exercise or eating habits. Janice reached her goals. Dale never did. I always hoped that I would one day work with Dale, once he fully understood that shortcuts don't work. Unfortunately, that day never came, and as far as I know, Dale is still looking for that miracle.

Remember that the desire to take a shortcut usually stems from not believing that you are capable of accomplishing your goals on your own. You are! Believe in yourself! Shortcuts are simply distractions from the one thing that can really change your life—working at it!

Change has to first take place *inside* of you. This is not true only when it comes to losing weight; it's true in all aspects of your life. By committing to Get with the Program, that's exactly what you're doing—starting the process of change. When you stop looking for the answer outside yourself, you'll elevate yourself. Above all, believe in yourself!

WRITTEN EXERCISE

Make a list of some of the shortcuts, gimmicks, diets, or trends that you've tried in the past that didn't work out. They don't have to pertain to only weight loss; they can relate to other areas of your life. Include an approximate time frame during which you tried them, and a summary of what happened in each case.

Date(s) _____

_____

_____

_____

_____

_____

Date(s) _____

_____

_____

_____

_____

_____

_____

Date(s) _____

_____

_____

_____

_____

_____

_____

Date(s) _____

_____

_____

_____

_____

3. Do you frequently use excuses to get yourself out of doing what it takes to reach your goals?

One of the things that I do for a living is help my clients overcome excuses. I've heard just about every one of them—except, of course, a good one!

"I don't have the time."

"I don't like to sweat."

"I feel claustrophobic when I'm out of breath."

"The rest of my family would never eat that."

"Then I'd have to shower before I go to work."

"I have to travel a lot in my line of work."

"My shins hurt when I do that."

"I have asthma."

"I get a rash when I do that."

"Then what do I do with all those sweaty clothes?"

"I'll start Monday."

"I'll start the first of the year."

"I'll focus on this next year."

I have to admit, I've become a little intolerant of excuses. In fact, if during initial consultations, I hear potential clients give three or more excuses why they can't make a necessary change in their lives, I won't work with them at that time. I'm not giving up on them; I'm simply making them wait until they're out of excuses, because that's what they need for their program to be successful. So many people just want to talk about changing. But when it comes right down to doing the hard work or making the tough decisions, they prefer to offer an excuse why they must continue living their lives just as they are. Don't be a victim of your own excuses. If you have excuses, you're not ready, plain and simple.

If you are afflicted with "chronic excuse syndrome," there's still hope. You must first recognize that you are using excuses to hold on to the life that you currently have. Then you must fully understand the consequences of the way you are choosing to live your life, including how it not only negatively affects you, but how it negatively affects others in your life. Accept that you've been avoiding these issues. When you are no longer satisfied defending your choices through excuses, and are willing to take responsibility for all of your choices—past, present, and future—you're ready to Get with the Program.

WRITTEN EXERCISE

Write down some of the excuses that you have used in the past for not doing something that would have improved your life. Be sure to include the dates you used these excuses, and place a check mark next to any that you have used in the past thirty days. Upon review and reflection, circle those that you now feel are without genuine merit and which ended up holding you back from something you really wanted to accomplish.

Date _____

Excuse: _____

_____

_____

_____

_____

Date _____

Excuse: _____

_____

_____

_____

_____

Date _____

Excuse: _____

_____

_____

_____

_____

_____

Date _____

Excuse: _____

_____

_____

_____

_____

_____

4. Are you often impatient with slow results?

Everyone is! But it still never ceases to amaze me how someone can gain weight over a period of, say, twenty or thirty years and expect dramatic weight loss results in a week or two. It just doesn't work that way! Losing weight the right way—through strengthening your body, gradually boosting your metabolism with exercise, and improving your eating habits—takes time. Powerful results in *any* area of your life are always best accomplished over time in small increments. Losing weight is no exception.

Most people who are successful at maintaining their motivation tend to take a long-term view of improving their life and their health. They tend to focus on the fact that they feel a little bit better today and are encouraged by knowing that they will feel even a little bit better tomorrow. That is exactly what I am asking you to do: Focus on feeling better and feeling better about yourself—today! Take the time to acknowledge and praise yourself each day that you stick with your chosen path to your goals, *especially* when results are slow. Also, as you make improvements, take the time to recognize them (such as small, positive changes in how your clothes fit). Above all, be sure to acknowledge the many ways that your life has improved since you Got with the Program. Make a list or keep a journal, but recognize your accomplishments! Take time to praise yourself each day that you "stick with it."

> I feel better.
>
> I sleep better.
>
> My clothes fit better.
>
> I'm not as stressed out.
>
> I'm gaining energy each day.
>
> I feel strong.
>
> I feel I can walk anywhere.
>
> I no longer get out of breath.
>
> I can do things that I couldn't before.
>
> I'm getting compliments on my appearance now.
>
> My skin looks better.
>
> I look healthier.

Impatience comes from focusing on negative thoughts. Results come from focusing on being happy today and constantly renewing your commitment to change and to improve the things that you can, one small step at a time.

WRITTEN EXERCISE

Write down things that make you happy and that you appreciate in your life—and how you can nurture them.

Appreciation _____

_____

_____

_____

_____

_____

Appreciation _____

_____

_____

_____

_____

_____

Appreciation _____

_____

_____

_____

_____

_____

5. Do you ever consider giving up when you experience minor setbacks?

Let me get this out in the open right now. You *will* experience setbacks—everyone does. The best way to look at setbacks is to see them as challenges and a natural part of your progress. Challenges add meaning to your life and represent opportunities for you to grow. If you can overcome your setbacks and reach your goals despite them, you have shown true strength, character, discipline, and determination. Your ultimate sense of accomplishment will be that much greater.

Many people I know use setbacks to let themselves off the hook. Consciously or unconsciously, they secretly want the opportunity to get out of the hard work of change or to confirm that they weren't meant to achieve what they set out to do. Don't be someone who waits for setbacks to occur; by doing so, you are really just using them as excuses to throw in the towel. Using setbacks in this way is a major reason that people return to their old habits and their previous way of life. Don't give in to it. Don't give up!

Don't let setbacks take away from your pride in the progress you've made. View these stumbling blocks as life's way of asking you: "How much do you really want this?" Be prepared to occasionally experience muscular soreness, blisters, body aches, colds, flu, disappointment, family commitments, work commitments, vacations, and lack of motivation.

Bet you can't wait to get started, huh?

Hey, it's life.

Needless to say, it helps to have a sense of humor—especially when you're trying to improve yourself and your life. The best advice I can give you is to keep a positive attitude. (It sounds like a cliché, but hey, sometimes clichés become clichés because they're true.) When it comes to maintaining weight loss, I can tell you that a positive attitude is one of the most important traits to possess. At the root of having a positive attitude is the core belief that you are fully capable of doing what it takes to reach your goals and the belief that you're going to continue doing what it takes through thick and thin. And that means for the rest of your life.

Before you really Get with the Program, program yourself for success. See yourself in your mind's eye completing and accomplishing your goals, and maintaining all of the necessary positive behaviors to insure your health and well-being for the rest of your life. Visualizing yourself reaching your goals will reinforce the need for you to shrug off "bad" days. Maintain a positive attitude and focus on today.

WRITTEN EXERCISE

Write about any times that you encountered setbacks in your life and overcame them. Include the approximate dates that these events occurred. Include how you felt when you triumphed over these obstacles.

Date _____

Setback: _____

_____

_____

Triumph: _____

_____

_____

Date _____

Setback: _____

_____

_____

Triumph: _____

_____

_____

Date _____

Setback: _____

_____

_____

Triumph: _____

_____

_____

Date _____

Setback: _____

_____

_____

Triumph: _____

_____

_____

Date _____

Setback: _____

_____

_____

Triumph: _____

_____

_____

6. Do you often procrastinate?

We've all been guilty of procrastination at one point or another. However, if this is a *frequent* pattern of behavior for you, it will have to be broken if you want results and you want them to last. Your success depends on your daily effort and recommitment to your goals.

Let's be honest: Procrastination is often really fear masked by laziness. Any time you want something or say that you want it, and you either don't take the proper steps to accomplish it or you act in direct opposition to it, you're being lazy as well as afraid. You may be afraid of failure, afraid of change, afraid of success, afraid of the unknown. For that matter, anything that holds you back can be directly traced back to the feeling of fear.

If procrastination is an element of your health and weight issues, you will need to focus extra hard on the true source of your fears. What is keeping you from starting a program to bring increased health and happiness into your life? What are you afraid of? Identify it. Once you do, you will conquer one of your greatest obstacles.

Get with the Program and break your personal cycle of procrastination.

You can do it.

Get started right now.

Commit to something that's important to you. Commit to this program today! Don't be afraid to be happy and healthy and strong. Read and sign the Get with the Program contract (see page 53) with yourself right now! Start a cycle of positive momentum by taking small steps toward your goals each day and feeling good about each of those steps that you take. Finish reading this book. Pick the day that you'll begin to exercise. Buy your athletic shoes. Buy your workout clothes. Rearrange your schedule to accommodate your exercise. Let the people in your life know that this program is important to you. Above all, honor your commitment to yourself.

WRITTEN EXERCISE

After you sign the Get with the Program contract with yourself, make a list of all the things that you need to do to begin fulfilling your commitment to this program (for example: purchasing workout clothing and shoes, deciding on which activities to add to your life, arranging for a baby-sitter, and so on), and include a start date for each.

Start date   **Task**

_____   _____

_____   _____

_____   _____

_____   _____

_____   _____

_____   _____

_____   _____

_____   _____

_____   _____

7. Are you afraid of change?

Change takes you from your comfort zone into the unknown. Change usually requires you to overcome fear; and while it's not always an easy thing to overcome, once you do, your life will change, and change for the better.

Fear of change can be paralyzing. It can freeze you in your tracks and delay you from getting what you want and deserve to have in your life. This type of fear often occurs with people who struggle with their weight. Many use their excess weight as an armor against change. This armor closes them off from the rest of the world.

SAFE BUT NOT SOUND

Holding on to extra weight may often serve as a person's unconscious anesthetic against stress, hurt, disappointment, pain, failure, and (sadly) even success, love, and romantic attention from potential suitors. It keeps many on the sidelines of life.

Being overweight helps make many fearful people feel as if they are invisible. This often makes the weight loss journey that much more difficult for some because as their weight begins to decrease so does their self-imposed protection from everyday life. Often they seek ways to sabotage themselves in order to return to the safety that their excess weight provides. If this is you, take heart. When you do find the courage to risk change and experience it in small doses, at your own rate, you're in for a powerfully wonderful, life-changing experience.

If you recognize how you've used fear to influence a decision that has held you back, you may wish you could rewrite the past. You can't. But you can make a decision to move forward now. Now is the best time to change your life! It's time to get out of your comfort zone and take some risks. It's definitely going to involve some effort. But you've gotten this far, and I'm sure you're ready to keep going.

In *Get with the Program*, you won't be asked to do anything that you're not capable of, and all of the challenges are accomplished on *your* timetable.

WRITTEN EXERCISE

Write down three instances in which you successfully overcame your fear of change. Include when each occurred, how you overcame the fear, and how the experience changed your life. If you believe you have subconsciously held on to your excess weight to keep a certain change from occurring in your life, identify those specific fears, then explain them and how and when they started. Once you do, you will begin to feel a surge of deep-healing relief as you get in touch with those inner feelings and let them out. Just start writing and let it flow.

Date _____

_____

_____

_____

_____

_____

Date _____

_____

_____

_____

_____

Date _____

_____

_____

_____

_____

Date _____

_____

_____

_____

_____

_____

Date _____

_____

_____

_____

_____

8. Do you typically choose immediate gratification over reaching your long-term goals?

Whether it was choosing those chocolates over fitting into a particular outfit or skipping a workout to go lie in the sun, everyone at one time or another has caved in to immediate gratification. If this is your theme song, however, it will make a successful weight loss program impossible because the process relies, in part, on your ability to give up temptations that are in front of you now for the benefit of your future well-being. In short, you must be willing at times to delay gratification.

Remember that no matter who you are or what your life is like, you'll need to make some sacrifices when it comes to this new commitment to your health and well-being. You are not only going to have to rearrange your life to some extent in order to free up the needed time, you will be doing something during that time that won't always be one of your favorite things to do—namely exercise! And the gratification that you'll receive from it certainly isn't immediate.

Needless to say, your willpower will be tested.

At those times, you should remind yourself of what your goals are and how important they are to you. You should also make a habit of picturing yourself reaching your goals and then reflecting on how gratifying that will be if you can just get past your moment of temptation. Surround yourself with reminders of what you want to accomplish. In a conspicuous place, hang an article of clothing that you one day would like to wear. Place the invitation to your high school reunion on your nightstand or desk. Do things that help you get past moments of temptation and that encourage you to focus on reaching your goals. Any time you're tempted to miss your exercise session or to eat something that you know is out of bounds, draw upon these things for strength.

Hmmmm . . .

potato chips now or a trim figure later?

When you're tempted to stray, you can also try writing down what it is you're giving up and what (in the future) you're getting in return. When you look at these choices in black and white, the choice starts to become at least a little bit easier.

Remember that you are not alone. Everyone wishes their results came more easily and more quickly, but results do eventually come to those who are patient and disciplined. What I'm asking you to do here is to *think differently* and to feel better about resisting temptation than you would about the fleeting pleasure of giving in to it. Start investing directly in yourself! Small sacrifices now will result in great returns in the future. It's the disciplined investor who shows the best results in the long run. If you can concentrate a little each day on your long-term goals, you will be successful!

Ultimately, willpower is the main ingredient in reaching your goals, but you can make it easier on yourself by building exercise and good eating habits into your lifestyle. You not only need to clear your schedule to accommodate your increased exercise during this phase, you must make exercise and good food choices as regular as brushing your teeth or taking a shower. *Your physical activity can no longer be negotiable!* From this time of your life on, remember that you need to move more to live more and eat more wisely to live more happily.

WRITTEN EXERCISE

Make a list of the things that you can do that will remind you of your long-term weight loss goal. This can include placing pictures of yourself or invitations to upcoming events in conspicuous places, displaying clothes that you'd like to wear: anything that keeps you focused on your goals. Once you make your list, write out a detailed plan about where you'll keep these things in view and how they'll be used in times of temptation.

List of reminders:

_____

_____

_____

_____

_____

Plan:

_____

_____

_____

_____

_____

9. Do you ever use family, relationship, or work obligations as an excuse not to take care of yourself?

I covered excuses earlier, but I wanted to devote some extra comments about the big three: family, relationship, and work obligations. This boils down to an issue of priorities. If you answered yes to this question, you need to make concern for your own health and well-being one of your top priorities—as it should be! (I'd love to see it be your number-one priority but let's definitely make it one of the top three.) Think of anything worthwhile that you've accomplished in your life, and try to tell me that you didn't make it one of your top priorities. It just doesn't work any other way.

From this point on, your health and well-being must be considered absolutely sacred. Your daily workout is also sacred. It is a gift you give yourself. Believe me, your career, family, and relationships with others (as well as your own self-esteem) will all benefit tremendously if you stay on track with this. You'll also set a terrific example for those in your life whom you really care about and who really care about you. I feel so strongly that this is exactly where most people fall off the wagon, I would recommend that if you're unsure whether you can make the commitment of time then you should consider holding off on starting the program until you are able to do so.

WRITTEN EXERCISE

Create an "I'm my own top priority" log. Starting now and for at least the next couple of weeks, simply jot down, in the spaces provided, each time you *avoid* letting family, relationship, or work obligations interfere with something you wanted to do for yourself. The emphasis here needs to be on the creative solutions you came up with that allowed you to accomplish what you wanted to do. Of particular interest should be any situations that you handle differently than you have in the past. Be sure to record the date that these occasions occur and the events surrounding each situation.

I'M MY OWN TOP PRIORITY

Date _____

_____

_____

_____

_____

Date _____

_____

_____

_____

_____

Date _____

_____

_____

_____

_____

Date _____

_____

_____

_____

_____

10. Are you afraid of disappointing others?

Whether you realize it or not, the fact that you're taking care of yourself will affect other people in your life. Some will be thrilled, others won't be so thrilled; but if you're overly concerned about disappointing someone else, you're wide open to failing in your efforts. There are at least three emotions that can come into play here: guilt, fear of disapproval, and fear that a relationship will be damaged or lost. These emotions can cause havoc to your program.

If you feel the least bit guilty about taking the time to exercise, eating healthy foods, or doing things for your overall health and happiness, I have three words for you: *Get over it!* Besides, only when you take care of yourself can you be of real help and value to anyone else.

———————————

caring about yourself and doing good things for yourself is not only your right, it's your responsibility.

———————————

The chances that you'll be challenged on your efforts are fairly good, whether it's someone being offended that you're not overindulging in a meal he prepared for you, someone trying to make you feel bad about turning her down to have a drink, or having to explain why you must meet someone a little later than he wished because of your workout. Eventually someone will be inconvenienced because you are standing up for yourself. Whatever the reason, get tough! You simply can't afford to worry about how taking care of yourself is going to disappoint someone else. Those who really care about you will not only understand but will be 100 percent behind you.

In addition to the guilt you may feel, it's quite possible to fear that someone will disapprove of your "self-indulgence." The extreme of this is when you fear that a relationship will be damaged or lost from your actions. These are irrational fears. Just ask yourself, "Who could possibly care about me and *not* want me to be happy and healthy?" If you really feel that you deserve to be happy and healthy, and that it's your right and responsibility to pursue your goals, then guilt, fear of disapproval, and fear that a relationship will be damaged or lost will no longer be issues for you.

Writing in a journal each day can help reinforce the importance of taking care of your needs and putting yourself first. Say it out loud, now: It's my right and my responsibility to care for myself. And believe it! When this becomes one of your core beliefs, the rest of the program becomes much easier.

The reactions of those close to you, such as your significant other, friends, relatives, colleagues, and acquaintances, may range from enthusiastic support to mild jealousy to outright sabotage. Efforts to sabotage you may be voiced as concern or attempts to make you feel guilty or uncomfortable. Sometimes these attempts are unconscious. Sometimes they are not.

"Have a little of this."

"Let's go out for a few drinks."

"You want some of this?"

"Come on, what do you mean you don't want seconds?"

"I made it especially for you."

"It won't hurt you just this once."

"You're looking too thin."

"I think you're just doing this to get attention from other people."

"What do you mean you have to exercise?"

"You can skip it just this once. Come on, we'll have fun."

"You've gotten so boring since you started this health kick."

You get the picture. Virtually everyone I have known who has lost a significant amount of weight has had someone in their life attempt to sabotage their efforts in some way. What this always boils down to is how *your* weight loss is going to affect *them*. Don't take acts of sabotage too personally. It's human nature for people to protect the relationship status quo. Remember that change is a challenge for everyone—even positive change, as you well know by now. This is usually the time for that honest conversation that's probably long overdue. Be firm but sympathetic to your saboteur's needs.

My advice is that before you get too far along in this process, get those close to you on board. Explain to them what it means to you to accomplish your goals and then ask them for their encouragement and support. They may even be inspired to Get with the Program themselves, but if not, at least they'll feel included in the process. Those who are close to you may need reassurance that your relationship with them will not be negatively affected. In particular, your spouse or significant other can be a critical factor in your success or failure. Their fear that you will leave them behind both figuratively and literally is a real and common problem. Again, make them feel included in the process and reassure them that achieving your goals is good for your relationship.

WRITTEN EXERCISE

Make a list of people in your life who may be most affected by your weight loss efforts. Once the list is complete, begin to communicate with each person about the importance of his support. Record when and where these conversations take place and any details about the person's reaction.

PEOPLE WHO MAY BE AFFECTED

Date _____

_____

_____

_____

_____

Date _____

_____

_____

_____

_____

Date _____

_____

_____

_____

_____

Date _____

_____

_____

_____

_____

11. Do you ever blame something or someone else for your inability to reach your goals?

If you answered yes to this question, you must look at whether or not you are taking full responsibility for your life. This is essential to making permanent changes and getting results. Pointing to external reasons for why your life has become and remains a certain way is much easier than realizing that you have control over your own life. We've all known people who have pointed to an unpleasant childhood, a bad marriage or relationship, or their less than fulfilling career as the cause for their unhappiness. They project the blame anywhere but on themselves by citing external causes. Projecting blame usually takes them farther from resolving anything.

Alice's Story

A couple of years back I had a client who asked me if it would be all right if she brought a friend to our workouts twice a week. She said her friend had always struggled with her efforts to lose weight and really needed some help. I told her that I thought it was a great idea.

Alice came to our next workout; she seemed quite pleasant. As time passed, Alice was visibly showing very good results; but about five weeks into her program, she started to miss at least one workout each week. She had mentioned that her mother-in-law had made some comments about her being away from home so much and that these comments really bothered her. On top of that, she had mentioned that her husband wasn't thrilled about the healthy dinners that were now being served. Soon after this conversation, her attendance was extremely sporadic. Most of the good results she had achieved were slipping away.

It seemed like an open and shut case of Alice trying to please everyone else in her life, as well as experiencing a little sabotage from those close to her. My client and I conspired. She would make sure, by hook or by crook, to get Alice to work out the next week, and I would confront Alice about her loss of commitment. When Alice showed up the next week, I asked her why her attendance had become so sporadic. She immediately became defensive and started mentioning everyone in her life, past and present, who was to blame for her inability to work out with us twice a week and for her inability to lose weight. She even implicated her dog!

Whoa! This was way beyond just wanting to please people or fearing their disapproval, this was blaming them for her lot in life. It was clear that Alice was not taking responsibility for her own decisions or her own life. The next workout, I talked to her privately about my concerns. It was an emotional discussion and

Alice admitted that she had blamed other people for her short-comings all her life.

While not all stories have happy endings, this one does. Alice reached her goal weight eight months after that talk. In addition, she claims that her relationships with her spouse, relatives, and friends have never been better, or more honest.

Alice took control by taking a good look at herself, her actions, and her issues. Alice Got with the Program by getting real with herself.

Taking responsibility means looking to *yourself* to create your own life. It means no longer blaming other people or things for who you are. Being successful with the weight loss process requires you to release all the external causes for your unhappiness, and then take it upon yourself to create your *own* happiness.

WRITTEN EXERCISE

List the three most important things that you want to accomplish in the year ahead. List all of the obstacles that are currently in your way of accomplishing these things. Then list the things that you can do to overcome these obstacles. Be sure to include exactly when you will initiate your plans.

Goals

1. _____

_____

2. _____

_____

3. _____

_____

Obstacles

_____

_____

_____

_____

_____

Solutions

_____

_____

_____

_____

_____

12. Do you ever feel that you don't deserve to be happy or successful?

If you're prone to sabotaging your own efforts or allowing anyone else to do so, it may be that deep down you really want your efforts to be doomed. There are a variety of reasons why you may do this, but typically the source stems from some type of fear. It could be fear of failure, fear of change, fear of loss, fear of disapproval, fear that you'll have to continue this life of constant effort, or even fear of success. But often at the root of this type of sabotage is the core belief that you're undeserving of happiness.

_____

Believing you are unworthy is the single greatest barrier to your success in achieving not only weight loss but anything worthwhile.

_____

Feeling unworthy is a more common trait than most people realize. It's even quite possible to consciously think that you deserve to be healthy and happy and unconsciously feel the opposite. If you are prone to self-sabotage (or allow others to sabotage your efforts) or you frequently notice that you derail your efforts just when you start showing results or are close to your goal, it's quite possible that you have a core belief that you are undeserving of happiness. Not only is this a common trait, for most people it's a very difficult obstacle to overcome.

Moving past this involves releasing your fears, both the fear that you really don't deserve to be happy and the fear of experiencing happiness. You can support this process by actively pursuing self-discovery techniques and enhancing your self-esteem. And this is exactly what Get with the Program is all about. I promise you that if you stick with the program, your sense of well-being will blossom and grow as you treat your body with the respect and the nurturing care it has always deserved. You can choose right now to pursue happiness and not to fear it. Be brave. And be happy.

WRITTEN EXERCISE

Write about the times that you've experienced success and/or happiness and then did something to sabotage the feeling or achievement. Include dates, if you can.

If you suspect that your core belief is that you don't deserve happiness, write an essay as to why you feel that you don't deserve it. Use the happiness journal below for this exercise. Frequently, when we see our arguments in writing, they are impossible to justify—even to ourselves! The sheer action of writing down your feelings will be a major step in your journey toward achieving well-deserved and earned health and happiness.

Date _____

_____

_____

_____

_____

_____

Date _____

_____

_____

_____

_____

Date _____

_____

_____

_____

_____

HAPPINESS JOURNAL

_____

_____

_____

_____

_____

_____

_____

_____

_____

_____

_____

_____

_____

_____

_____

_____

_____

_____

_____

_____

_____

_____

_____

_____ (date completed) _____

Phase One Written Exercise

The final exercise in Phase One is for you to reflect on and write about *why you've failed in the past with other fitness and weight loss plans.* Use the space below to write an essay detailing what didn't work and why. Write about the emotional reasons for your failure. Were any of the twelve issues above to blame? Describe which of the old thought patterns you will now need to get rid of or change in order to successfully Get with the Program.

FINAL ESSAY

Date _____

_____

_____

_____

_____

_____

_____

_____

_____

_____

_____

_____

_____

_____

_____

_____

_____

_____

_____

_____

Get with the Program is about changing your behavior, and changing your behavior requires you to change the way you think. It may be hard work to exercise regularly and make positive eating changes, but the real challenge is to take a good, hard, honest look at yourself and summon up the courage to make permanent, positive changes in the way you think and behave. While this is one of the toughest things you could possibly do, it can also be one of the most rewarding and life changing!

• • •

~

*G*et with the *P*rogram

*C*ontract with *M*yself

I hereby pledge to exercise in accordance with my Get with the Program requirements, to nourish my body with the quantity and quality of nutrients that will make me flourish, and to dedicate my efforts to elevate and care for myself to the best of my ability.

_____ Day of _____ 20 _____

_____

(signature)

I congratulate you for making it this far. Now invest in yourself by signing the Get with the Program Contract with Myself (see page 53) and posting it on your refrigerator. It will help motivate you along your journey.

THE TRUTH ABOUT YOUR WEIGHT

It all seems so simple. You're trying to lose weight, you jump on the scale, you see you've dropped two pounds, and you feel good about yourself. Two days later you jump on the same scale, you see you've gained a pound, and this triggers an emotional crisis! What if the entire process of weighing yourself was one big practical joke? Well, in a way, it is!

Let me explain. In the first scenario, let's say you lost four pounds of water, gained three pounds of fat, and lost a pound of muscle. When you jumped on the scale, it would read that you lost two pounds. The chances are that you felt pretty good about yourself, even though the reality is that you *gained three pounds of fat.* You just didn't know it. In the second scenario, you've lost four pounds of fat and gained five pounds of water. The scale read that you gained a pound, when the truth is that you *lost four pounds of unwanted body fat.* Your reaction would probably be one of disappointment.

By understanding the shortcomings of the bathroom scale as well as a little bit about the science behind how your body gains and loses weight, you can avoid the emotional roller coaster that weighing yourself can put you through. In fact, frustration from the lack of results and erratic fluctuations in weight are very common causes for people to give up their weight loss program. This is exactly why I want you to learn everything you need to know about your body weight, so you can avoid this frustration. Let's start at the beginning.

The first type of body weight is *water weight.* This refers to the weight of all the water in your body, including water found within your bloodstream, your digestive tract, as well as the water that is within all of the cells found in the various types of tissue that make up your body.

The second type of weight is *fat weight.* This refers to the weight of all the fat that is found within your body. Fat is not only found in your fat-deposit sites (such as your thighs, the back of your arms, or your abdomen), it also surrounds and is within the vital organs of your body. It's found within your muscles and, unfortunately, within the walls of your arteries and veins, as well as within the heart muscle itself. Lipids, which are basic building blocks of fat, are found within virtually every cell of your body. Fat is the one tissue in your body that contains very little water.

Lastly, there's *lean weight.* This refers to the weight of everything that is not water or fat, such as your muscles, hair, bones, cartilage, and other tissues.

When you lose weight, you can lose either water, fat, or lean weight. The loss of lean weight is something you *definitely* don't want to happen. One of the side effects of the loss of lean weight (usually muscle) is a decreased metabolism. The loss of lean weight occurs when you're inactive. It also occurs when you severely restrict the amount of calories that you consume—such as when you are dieting. The loss of lean weight can also be an occurrence of the aging process, with the most pronounced losses coming from your muscles and your bone mass, the latter of which is known as osteoporosis. Exercise in general is effective, but strength training in particular has been shown to be one of the most effective ways to prevent the loss of muscle as well as bone mass. Gains in muscle weight can occur at almost any age with the use of strength training exercises.

The loss of water weight occurs constantly through the metabolic processes of sweating and urination. When you lose excessive amounts of water weight, you become dehydrated. This is also something that you don't want to happen. Dehydration is a very subtle and common problem. When you're dehydrated, most of the important processes that are performed by your body become less effective, including the metabolism of fat. Believe it or not, most people are walking around dehydrated to some degree.

Your body has the ability to store a lot of extra water, especially when you drink a lot of it and are very active. You will need to be prepared for significant gains in your water weight when you first begin Get with the Program. In the first four or five weeks, the increase in your water weight will probably hide the fact that you are losing fat. Please don't be frustrated. Be patient. This means that good things are happening.

When you say that you want to lose weight, what you really mean is that you want to lose fat. The loss and gain of body fat occurs continually. In general, when your total energy requirements (calories expended) exceed your total energy consumed (calories eaten), your body breaks down body fat for energy, which, in turn, leads to fat weight loss. The reverse is also true. If you consume more energy (calories) than you expend, you'll store this excess energy as body fat.

You may not realize it, but your body automatically protects itself against losing too much fat too quickly. This protection mechanism exists to guard your stored energy (fat) and to protect you against starvation. What you might not be aware of is that even if you are absolutely diligent with your eating and exercise habits and have a favorable metabolism, the greatest amount of fat weight that you can lose in a week is about three pounds. Now, if you've ever been on a severely calorie-restricted diet, you might remember losing up to ten pounds in a given week—maybe even more. This lost weight was a combination of water, lean weight, and *no more than three pounds of fat*—with most of the loss coming from your water weight. This is especially true if your diet was of the high-protein, low-carbohydrate type. Losing weight through dieting often leads to dehydration, which, ironically, lowers your body's ability to burn fat. This is not what you want to happen and is just one more reason that you should not restrict your calories too much, especially in lieu of exercising. It's also why a *slower* weight loss is to your advantage.

You can start to see why jumping on that scale certainly doesn't give you the whole picture. You'll soon learn about erratic fluctuations and plateaus in your weight that are due to a variety of factors, which will further complicate matters. So how do you determine if you're making progress?

To Weigh or Not to Weigh?

If I had my way, I would view the weight of my clients without them knowing what that weight was. This is because it can provide me with some helpful information, but only because I know how to properly interpret it; and it would protect my clients from the seesaw of emotions that go along with weighing themselves regularly. However, most people who wish to lose weight can't avoid the temptation to jump on the scale. They need immediate gratification, even if they risk the disappointment of the scale informing them that they have gained weight—or not lost any weight. For some people this disappointment can even lead to the end of their weight loss program. Don't let it happen to you.

As for what *you* should do, weigh yourself right now and record this weight in the information section of your Get with the Program Journal at the end of Phase One (see page 88). Then you won't weigh yourself again until you begin Phase Three. This is because, particularly in the first two phases, you will be gaining water weight, and these extra pounds of water will hide the fact that you're losing body fat. Starting in Phase Three, you will weigh yourself only once a week, and even then you'll need to fully understand the shortcomings of the scale. Starting right now, however, pay close attention to how your clothes fit—this is the best overall way to gauge the loss of body fat. Why? Because fat takes up *considerably* more space than water. For the most part, if your clothes are fitting more loosely, you're losing body fat. If they're fitting more tightly, you're gaining body fat.

In Phase Three, when you combine the correctly interpreted information that the scale gives you with how your clothes fit, you should have a good idea if you're gaining or losing fat.

When you finally do start weighing yourself, be sure to always:

1. Use the same scale.
2. Weigh yourself only one day per week, at approximately the same time on the same day each week. (Monday mornings work well since this may prevent you from overindulging throughout the weekend.)
3. Be consistent with what you wear.

By understanding what's happening to your body and your weight, you will be able to determine if you're on the right path, and you'll avoid the frustration when the scale is not budging or—even worse—when it moves higher. Trust me, at some point this will happen! Everyone experiences weight loss plateaus and sudden weight increases. It's simply part of the weight loss process.

The Many Ways That Your Body Weight Can Be Erratic and Unpredictable

Your weight can go up, go down, or plateau for a number of reasons. Some fluctuations you have control over and some you do not. You should become familiar with everything that affects your body weight so that you can know what's taking place when you weigh yourself and avoid the frustration when the scale is not participating in your weight loss program.

WATER FLUCTUATIONS

Be forewarned that when you first become active or increase the amount and intensity of your exercise, you will retain extra water. Gaining this extra water weight can be disheartening and, as I mentioned before, has caused many people to give up their exercise programs. The truth is that gaining this extra water weight is a very good sign.

As you become more active and drink more water, your muscles will act like sponges and will immediately become more fully hydrated. In addition, you may also add a little new muscle, which in turn will store even more water. The more active you are, the more glycogen (a stored carbohydrate) your muscles will retain. Each gram of glycogen stores an additional 2.5 to 3 grams of water. Finally, the better shape you're in, the more water is stored within your bloodstream. This additional water weight gain can be significant and is most pronounced when you increase your level of fitness. This explains why physically fit individuals store considerably more water within their bodies than unfit individuals. This also explains how a very fit person can weigh much more than their appearance would suggest.

When you exercise regularly, you're sending the message to your body that water needs to be stored in relatively large quantities. Your body responds by finding creative ways to store this additional water. The fitter you become, the higher your percentage of water weight will be, and the lower your percentage of body fat. Don't let this additional water weight frustrate you. It's a good sign! It means that your metabolism is increasing as well as your potential to burn fat. That's why I especially like to see my new clients put on this initial water weight; it usually means that good things are about to happen—that is, as long as they remain patient through the first four to six weeks.

In addition to the initial water weight gain that you'll experience when you become more active, your body has various water cycles that influence the retention and release of water weight. There are daily, weekly, monthly, and even seasonal water cycles. These cycles occur for a variety of complex reasons, and they are not all fully understood. There are also times when these cycles converge to reach their respective highs, at which time you'll experience a significant increase in your water weight and, consequently, your total weight. It's at these times when you must reassure yourself that as long as you are consistently "on the program," there will be a gradual reduction in your body fat—even if the scale doesn't confirm it! By the same token, there will be times that the various water cycles converge at a low point, resulting in your body's retaining less water. This will lead to a decrease in your total body weight. This is also somewhat of an illusion and should not cause you to become overconfident.

It all comes down to trust—trust in yourself! As long as you are patient and believe you are doing the best thing for yourself and that you deserve the results you desire, *those good results will happen!*

Another cause of water retention is the result of too much salt in your diet. It is also the consequence of consuming monosodium glutamate (MSG), which is a common food additive that contains sodium (salt). This weight is temporary and will be lost as soon as your body eliminates the sodium. Many quick-fix diets will recommend that you completely avoid salty foods. A primary reason for this is so that you'll appear to be successful on the diet when you weigh yourself, regardless of whether you are actually losing fat weight or water weight. Keep in mind that although your body needs a minimum amount of sodium, most people get more than enough by eating a balanced diet (without adding salt to their food). *Individuals who need to be on a salt-restricted diet due to high blood pressure or other health complications should consult with their physician for guidelines regarding salt consumption.*

Caffeine, on the other hand, is a diuretic and causes your body to rid itself of water; consuming too much caffeine can lead to dehydration. Therefore, foods and beverages that contain caffeine (such as coffee, tea, chocolate, and certain sodas) should be kept to a minimum. Also, keep in mind that caffeine is often present in many quick-fix weight loss supplements and diet drinks—for the obvious reason.

Certain vitamins, nutritional supplements, and medications can also cause the body to retain or release water and will affect your body weight. Your physician or pharmacist can give you specific information on the water-retention effects of any substance that you may be taking.

Most women experience a temporary increase of water weight just prior to their menstrual period; water weight can cause bloating and may affect the way a woman's clothes fit temporarily. By the time a woman's period is finished, the weight has usually disappeared. A great many people experience a significant increase in water weight just before they drop fat weight. Why this happens is not fully understood. One explanation relates this temporary water weight gain to a person's monthly water cycle. Yet another theory states that when you lose fat, which takes up a relatively large amount of space, your body retains water to temporarily fill that space until your body can accommodate the change (I'll talk about this in a little more detail later). Regardless of why, this happens. It's just one more way your body can play a practical joke. Don't let it get the better of you.

Water weight gain is commonly responsible for the scale not budging—or even moving higher. Remember that each time you improve your level of fitness your body holds more water. Don't worry about it. In reality, increasing your water weight is a sign that good things are about to happen. Water fluctuations happen to everyone and are nothing to be concerned about unless you let them affect your emotions. If you suspect that you're retaining water, just examine how your clothes fit. If, despite an increase in your weight, your clothes fit about the same or even more loosely, water is probably to blame. When you lose weight the right way, by being active, the rules change a bit. It's very common to be losing fat but gaining weight. As frustrating as this can be, my advice is to simply focus on how good you feel, how your clothes fit, and the other positive changes that are happening to you.

Seasonal Weight Gain

Have you ever noticed that you carry more weight in the winter months? (This may be why so many of us begin our serious fitness programs in January.) There are several reasons for this. For one, whether it's out of habit or due to the inclement weather, we move less in the winter. When we spend more time indoors, we tend to have fewer choices of activities, which, in turn, can lead to eating more. On top of this, most of the "power eating" holidays occur in the colder months. Finally, there actually may be a biological mechanism that causes us to gain weight in the winter. And while this is not 100 percent proven or understood, it does make sense. Perhaps your body is "programmed" to store more fat in the winter to ensure you're insulated against the cold and won't starve if there's a shortage of food. Most health professionals will tell you to avoid overeating at holidays and to keep your activity level consistent throughout the winter months. I would certainly agree with this advice. However, I also don't believe that your weight was meant to stay exactly the same all year round. I think you should allow your weight to fluctuate in a range with which you're comfortable and that takes into account your body's natural cycles. Otherwise, you're constantly fighting nature and driving yourself crazy.

I know my eating stays fairly consistent all year long, as does my activity level. However, I'm always five or six pounds heavier in the winter months—and this pattern has occurred for as long as I can remember. Oh, yes, except for that one year when I developed a severe craving for pecan pie, which lingered well after the holiday season. Pecan pie being one of the most calorically dense foods on the planet, those five or six pounds became ten that year!

Typically, though, these five or six pounds feel very comfortable to me.

In fact, I'd probably miss them if they didn't show up one winter, though I'm also glad to see them go in the late spring. I can't imagine being bothered by this seasonal weight gain to the point of exercising obsessively or overly restricting my eating during the holidays. I strongly recommend that you ignore moderate seasonal weight fluctuations and just continue being active and eating right. Seasonal weight gain is natural, as well as temporary, and there is no need to adjust what you're doing to respond to it. If your seasonal weight gain is higher than, say, eight pounds (like it was the year of my pecan pie debacle!), especially if this is more than you've experienced in the past, it's time to look at some other explanation for the gain.

Aftereffects When You Quit Smoking

Quitting smoking cigarettes may be the single best thing you can do for yourself.

I won't spend a lot of time lecturing about how smoking accelerates nearly every disease process known to man, including heart disease and various forms of cancer—I'm sure you're aware of that. But what you might *not* be aware of is how smoking places a ceiling on your level of fitness and can make *permanent* weight loss more difficult.

Many smokers have a desire to quit someday. However, when they actually do, they have a good chance of regaining any weight they may have lost up until that point. The average weight gain is between eight and fifteen pounds. The frustration of gaining back weight that was lost often causes them to start smoking all over again. While smoking raises your metabolism and therefore allows you to maintain a lower body weight in the short term, the long-term effects of this addictive habit always negatively affect your health, your level of fitness, and your motivation to improve either. Smoking lowers the amount of oxygen that is carried in your blood. This significantly inhibits your ability to both exercise and, ultimately, burn fat.

Just remember that smokers who are overweight and continue to smoke tend to remain overweight. Ex-smokers who are inactive also tend to remain or become overweight. But ex-smokers who consistently exercise have the best chance of both remaining off cigarettes and keeping their weight under control.

The best time to quit smoking is *now*, when you first Get with the Program. The act of exercising significantly decreases your urge to smoke. Exercising will also reduce the negative effects of stress in your life, primarily through the release of endorphins, which are natural painkillers produced by your body. This effect will further curb the urge to smoke. In addition, you now know that it is common to gain a few pounds of water when you first begin exercising, so you will be psychologically prepared for an initial weight gain at the beginning of the program. Don't fool yourself into thinking you'll give up smoking after you've lost a certain amount of weight. You'll probably be less willing to risk a sudden weight gain at that time. The bottom line is that you should make your plan to quit smoking now and stick to it.

BIOLOGICAL ADJUSTMENTS

Keep in mind that you need a certain amount of body fat to survive. Body fat protects your internal organs, insulates you from the cold, is an important source of stored vitamins and nutrients, and provides you with your primary source of stored potential energy. Therefore, when you begin to lose body fat too quickly, certain biological mechanisms are triggered to protect you. We don't completely understand how these fail-safe protections work, but we do know that from time to time your body needs to "take a breather" from losing weight. Once your body has adjusted to the changes you are making, it will go on its merry way, losing fat.

If at any point in the program you find that you've just stopped losing weight, there's a good chance that this is due to one of these biological adjustments. Be patient and continue with what you're doing. If the plateau in your weight continues for three or four weeks, you may have hit what is called a "real plateau."

Learning the difference between biological adjustments, water fluctuations, and hitting a real plateau is a skill— one that you can learn with just a little practice.

Realizing Your Set Point—When You Hit a Real Plateau

Sometimes you stop losing body fat for a period of time or it increases slightly. If you have ruled out all of the above explanations, you've probably hit a real plateau.

You see, you actually "defend" a certain percentage of body fat. By *de-*

fend I mean that given your genetics, your average daily activity, what and how much you eat, and the way you exercise, your body tightly regulates the amount of body fat that you maintain and keeps it within a certain range. If you don't change anything that you're currently doing (such as increase your level of exercise), you'll remain at more or less this level of body fat. In other words, you've realized your set point. Think of your set point as the setting on your body fat "thermostat." Each setting corresponds to the total amount of body fat that your body will maintain. Every time you make an adjustment to your thermostat by changing your exercise or eating habits, you change the setting. Increase the amount of exercise you perform, and you maintain a lower percentage of body fat. Cut out certain unhealthy foods, and, again, you maintain a lower percentage of body fat. But the important part about knowing when you've reached a real plateau (assuming that you want further results) is that it signals when it's time to add more exercise or move to the next phase of the program, or both. The key is to know when you've reached a real plateau, as opposed to one of the many other reasons why your body fat may have ceased to decrease.

So when have you officially hit a real plateau? First of all, don't even start the clock ticking until the initial weight gain due to water is behind you. This can take up to six weeks or even more for some people. (This is one of the reasons that I don't want you to weigh yourself in the first two phases of the program. To officially consider yourself at a real plateau, you need to have begun losing weight in the first place!) If you have begun to consistently lose weight and your weight loss stops for at least three weeks and you can rule out all of the other explanations we've talked about previously, the chances are that you've hit a real plateau. If you want to lose more, you'll need to add a little more exercise to your week. Now, I'll be the first to admit that three weeks is an arbitrary amount of time, but I think it is a valid reference point to begin evaluating where you stand and whether you need to make some changes in your program. Keep in mind that most water fluctuations are temporary, lasting only two or three days, and, for the most part, they are somewhat predictable once you learn your unique water patterns. I'm confident that within a few months you'll be able to determine the difference between when you're retaining water and whether you've hit a real plateau (and therefore realized your set point). But you must be patient through those first few months! Base everything on how you feel overall and how your clothes are fitting.

If losing weight is your primary goal, reaching a real plateau will probably not be something to which you're looking forward. This requires a change in how you think. Reaching a *real plateau* is exactly what you need to tell you if you're making progress. If you continue to show results, even if they are slow, continue what you're doing and enjoy the ride down before making any changes! Once you begin Phase Two and you are ready for further results, simply increase the amount of weekly minutes that you exercise, or if you're ready for the next phase—move up!

Margaret's Story

I met Margaret close to a year ago. The first day I started working with her I learned that she was forty-eight years old, she felt that she had been overweight her entire life, she was postmenopausal, she took not one but *two* medications that made weight loss more difficult, she never really participated in a structured exercise program, and she had tried virtually every diet known, but was currently not dieting. She also, for the most part, ate healthful foods; the only change to her eating habits she would eventually need to make was that she would need to eliminate her late night eating and she might have to reduce the total amount of food she consumed at some point in the future. Given all I had learned about Margaret, I knew that her weight loss would be slow and that she would need to be patient.

The years of dieting and general lack of exercise had taken their toll on Margaret's metabolism. Our first order of business would be to raise it, so I outlined an exercise program for her. She quickly asked me what she should be eating and I told her not to change anything yet. This surprised her. She began to exercise and quickly put on five pounds (of water). After three weeks she suggested that it must be time to modify her eating. I reinforced that her recent weight gain was in fact water and she should continue with just the exercise. After the fourth week, Margaret had lost three pounds. She was very excited about her weight loss as well as her ability to work so much harder. When she asked again if it was time to change her eating habits, I said no.

For the next three months, Margaret's weight followed a consistent pattern. It would first go up about three or four pounds, and then it would drop five or six pounds. Each time it would go up she would ask if it was time to "take a look at her eating" and each time I would say no. Eventually, Margaret hit what I felt was a real plateau—it took nearly five months to occur. Besides slightly increasing the amount of time she exercised, she needed to stop eating at least two hours before she went to bed. In addition, she would need to stop her habit of waking up in the middle of the night and having a snack. Gradually she did it, and her weight starting moving back down.

Eight months into her program, Margaret stopped losing weight again. She was convinced that now was the time her overall diet would need to be overhauled. But she was traveling a lot and had not been as consistent with her program while she was on the road. I convinced her to be concerned only about being consistent with her exercise and avoiding the late night eating. On renewing her commitment, she began losing weight again. She is now almost one year into her program, and what she eats during and in between meals has not changed from when she first began. Nevertheless, she continues to consistently drop about a pound a week.

Even after boosting her metabolism, Margaret was not capable of losing much more than a pound of body fat in any given week, so for her to be overly aggressive with her exercise and overly restrictive with her eating would have only made her tired and hungry, and inevitably would have caused her to quit.

Most people can realistically expect only one or two pounds of fat loss per week. Maybe once your metabolism is in high gear you could lose three pounds of fat in a week, but that's only if everything else, such as your eating and your exercise, is perfect—and it rarely is. The point is that slow, methodical weight loss is what you want for long-term results. It's all about increasing your metabolism and then allowing it to work for you, not against you. And remember, as long as your clothes are fitting better and you're experiencing other positive results, don't make any changes, even if the results are slower than you'd like.

Your Metabolism

The most dramatic changes to your body are going to occur due to changes in your metabolism. Rev up your metabolism and you'll lose body fat. Allow your metabolism to drop and your body fat increases—it's that simple.

What exactly is metabolism? It's the rate that your body burns calories. Many people make the mistake of thinking it's simply the *amount* of calories your body burns, but the key word here is *rate*. The rate of calories that your body burns can change, depending on what it is that you're doing. If you are sleeping, your metabolism will be burning calories at a relatively slow rate. This rate is often referred to as your resting, or basal, metabolic rate. Even though you may be asleep, you still need to burn calories for the basic functions of your body, such as breathing, maintaining your nervous system, and performing any digestion system functions. All these functions slow down when you're asleep. Once you wake up, so do all the functions that your body performs; this raises your metabolism. When you begin your basic daily activities, your metabolism increases further to meet your increased energy demands.

During exercise, your metabolism increases in direct proportion to the amount and intensity of your exercise. This is why your metabolism increases *immediately* in response to your activity level when you are exercising. But did you know that you can also make more permanent changes to your total metabolism and elevate it all twenty-four hours, each day of your life? This can be accomplished by aerobically exercising regularly. That is one of the secrets to making dramatically positive changes to your body!

How do you know if your metabolism is changing? Unfortunately, since metabolism refers to a rate of burning calories, there is no way to measure it directly. However, there are subtle cues that will tell you that it's changing. First of all, it has to increase *while* you're exercising; that's a given. Over time, as you gradually increase the amount and intensity of exercise that you're capable of doing, you can assume that your metabolism is increasing. But you will also notice a change in the way you perspire. When your metabolism increases, you will not only perspire more during exercise, but you will begin perspiring sooner into your workout. This is solid evidence that your metabolism is changing. Finally, as your clothes fit more loosely, you can conclude that this reflects an increased metabolism, especially when this occurs before you've reduced the amount of calories that you are consuming.

What Should Your Goal Weight Be?

I guess it's human nature to want to have a specific goal weight to focus on when you start a weight loss program. So how do you determine what that goal weight should be?

Well, you could consult one of the many charts or indexes that give you recommendations on what your weight should be based on your age, height, and frame size. Or you could go to a place that performs body fat analysis, get tested, then compare your results to established guidelines. (Unfortunately, for the most part these methods are inaccurate.) Or you could remember what your weight was when you were happy with it and base your goal weight on that. Except that times change. Your body changes. You may have gained muscle or water. You may have even gotten taller, or shorter. For a variety of reasons, it may not be appropriate for you to be the same weight that you were in, say, high school.

---

*Let me suggest something: Don't have a goal weight
at this time. Let it evolve as your body does.*

You're about to gain water weight and perhaps just a little bit of muscle weight. Your body will go through a variety of changes. It would be almost impossible to predict at this time what weight will be perfect (and realistic) for you months from now. You simply don't need a goal weight right now. I believe way too much is made about what you "should" weigh. On top of everything else, obsessing about reaching such an arbitrary goal keeps you from focusing on being happy today, which in the scheme of things is much more important.

THE TRUTH ABOUT DRINKING MORE WATER

Fact: There is a 75 percent chance that as you read this you are dehydrated. That's right! Seventy-five percent of all people don't drink enough water. The good news is that if you are one of them, you can hydrate yourself starting right now. So pour yourself a tall glass of clean, fresh water and read on about how drinking enough water can help you lose weight and make you much healthier overall.

Fact: Of all of the nutrients that we need to live and breathe and function healthily, water is the most essential. When you don't consume enough water, virtually every function that your body performs is compromised. This includes the important functions of digestion and fat metabolism. There's no doubt that by your being fully hydrated, all of the wonderful changes that you're about to make will work more effectively for you. You need to start drinking enough water now, even before you begin to elevate your metabolism with aerobic exercise.

Fact: Between 60 and 70 percent of your body weight is water, and you lose a lot of it each day through normal bodily processes. This lost water needs to be replaced if you're going to function at your best. Take a look below at the amazing benefits of water:

- **Your metabolism functions better when you're fully hydrated.** A strong metabolism requires a lot of water to be stored within your body. Water drives all the chemical reactions that are needed to burn calories both at rest and during exercise.
- **Your digestion is improved when you drink enough water.** Dehydration can lead to incomplete digestion, which in turn may prevent you from getting necessary nutrients, such as vitamins and minerals. These deficiencies can trigger unnecessary eating in order to receive a nutrient that your body needs.
- **Water fills you up.** By drinking enough water you can curb your appetite. Water tends to fill you up, which makes you less prone to overeating. A great idea is to have a tall glass of water about a half hour before each meal.
- **When you're dehydrated, you eat more.** When you're dehydrated, your body signals you to eat, when all it really requires is water. I call this effect "artificial hunger." Your body does the same thing for a variety of other nutritional needs as well. For example, when you're low on sodium, you crave foods that are salty. All you really need is the sodium without all the extra calories that come along with, say, the big soft pretzel that looks so tempting. This can also occur when your body needs particular vitamins or minerals. This is why it's so important to eat a well-balanced diet; when all of your nutritional needs are met, including your need for water, you'll be much less prone to food cravings and, therefore, overeating.
- **Your exercise is much more effective if you're fully hydrated.** Soon you'll be aerobically exercising and challenging your body on a regular basis. If you want that exercise to have its maximum effect on your metabolism, you'll need as much water as possible stored within your body so that the increased metabolic demands of exercise can be met. You'll also need additional water so that the important function of cooling your body through sweating can effectively take place. The bottom line

here is that if you're not fully hydrated before you start exercising, you'll do less work, burn less calories, and improve your metabolism to a lesser degree. Get into the habit of having a glass of water thirty minutes before you work out. And always be sure to meet your daily water quota. In Phase One, this quota is at least six full eight-ounce glasses—no less!

- **The more active you are, the fitter you become and the more water you need.** Whenever you're more active, your muscles soak up a lot more water. (This is another reason why you're going to need even more water than you usually drink.) In addition, you'll probably be adding some new muscle weight. Because muscle consists of more than 70 percent water, you'll need extra water for this extra muscle. Remember: The more fully hydrated muscles that you have in your body, the more potential "fat burners" you'll have working for you. Keep in mind that the entire process of becoming leaner is not only a process of losing body fat and gaining active muscle, but also a process of gaining water.

  Active muscles not only store more water, they store more glycogen. Glycogen is a form of carbohydrate that is stored in your muscles. Along with fat, it is used as an energy source when you exercise. The more fit you become, the more glycogen is stored within your muscles. This allows you to work at higher levels of exercise, which will help you become even fitter. Remember that every gram of glycogen within your body holds about 2.5 to 3 grams of water.

Your Self-Watering Instructions

In Phase One of the program, you will be drinking a *minimum* of 6 eight-ounce glasses of water each day. In Phase Two of the program, when you begin to become more active, your water requirement will be a minimum of 7 eight-ounce glasses of water each day. In Phase Three, you'll be exercising more and getting fitter, and you will need a minimum of 8 eight-ounce glasses of water each day. Finally, in Phase Four, you'll be exercising more and at higher levels; therefore, I want you to drink a minimum of 9 eight-ounce glasses of water each day. And I'm talking about plain, old-fashioned water. Sparkling water can have a diuretic effect, so it doesn't count. Even though other beverages, such as soda and coffee, contain water, they also don't count. Neither do foods that you eat, regardless of whether or not they have a high water content. Remember: Your water requirement is over and above the water that you get from other foods and beverages you consume. While some of these other sources may help you overcome dehydration, their consumption is factored into your overall daily requirement.

I also want you to get out of the habit of drinking water only when you're thirsty. Our thirst mechanism is flawed. By the time you experience thirst, your body is already in a state of dehydration. Even when your thirst is satisfied, you still may be dehydrated. It's important to drink water throughout the day, and it's best to drink only 1 or 2 eight-ounce glasses at any given sitting. This will help you to spread your water consumption over the course of the day, rather than drinking your eight glasses all at once. When you drink large quantities of water all at once, you stimulate your body to rid itself of water. Also, try not to drink your water too late in the evening, otherwise you'll find yourself waking up throughout the night!

Just a Few Tips to Keep You Hydrated

- Each time you reach for a beverage other than water, ask yourself if water would do the trick instead. You will be surprised at the number of times you're really just trying to quench your thirst.
- Alcohol dehydrates you, so you should limit the amount of alcohol you consume. (You will be actively limiting the amount of alcohol you consume during Phase Two, but it doesn't hurt to start a little early!)
- Caffeine is a strong diuretic. You should limit the amount of caffeine you consume. For example, if you drink tea or iced tea, try herbal tea.
- Purchase one of the many types of water filters for your home. Filtering tap water not only improves the taste of your water but also takes out any impurities and is less costly than purchasing bottled water.
- Make water available to yourself at all times. Carry a bottle of water around with you. Keeping water constantly with you will cause you to drink more of it. You'll reach your daily requirement, one sip at a time!
- Try drinking a glass of water shortly after you wake up. Have a glass before your workout. You'll be thirsty right afterwards, so have two more. Have another glass about a half hour before your lunch. Now you've already had five glasses, and it's not even lunchtime!
- Be aware that if you're trying to kick the smoking habit or limit your alcohol consumption, being fully hydrated has been shown to help these two worthy efforts tremendously!

PREPARING YOUR BODY TO EXERCISE:
BECOMING FUNCTIONALLY FIT

We were made to move, and when we don't, our quality of life is significantly lowered, whether it's by excessive weight gain, by the loss of bone mineral, by the loss of muscle, or through one of the many hypokinetic diseases that range from headache to heart disease. So in addition to increasing your daily activity by hiding the remote control, taking long walks after dinner, and using the stairs instead of the elevator, now is the time for you to begin to learn how to exercise properly.

It's time to give up the excuses and lace up your sneakers!

Obtaining Medical Clearance

You should always consult your physician before you start an exercise program. It's also a good idea to have a checkup prior to beginning Get with the Program. And that checkup should at the very least include your:

- blood pressure
- total cholesterol
- LDL cholesterol
- HDL cholesterol
- blood sugar reading

There is a place to record these values for your records in the Get with the Program Journal beginning on page 88.

What Is Fitness?

This seems like a straightforward question, but the truth is it's not. There are really different types of fitness.

Functional fitness refers to your ability to safely and effectively perform routine movements and exercise. In Phase One, we're going to emphasize your functional fitness, using exercises that will improve your flexibility, balance, and coordination, as well as the muscular strength and endurance of your abdomen, your back, the stabilizing muscles of your shoulders, and your lower legs.

Cardiovascular fitness refers to the ability of your heart, lungs, and arteries to deliver oxygen (which is carried in the blood) to working muscles *and* your muscles' ability to use that oxygen to perform aerobic work over a particular period of time. Your cardiovascular fitness is improved primarily through aerobic exercises. We're going to emphasize the improvement of your cardiovascular fitness starting in Phase Two of your program.

Then there's *muscular fitness.* Your muscular fitness refers to your muscular strength, muscular power, and muscular endurance. These are all important qualities that will be enhanced for the most part through the use of strength, or weight, training exercises. Your muscular fitness will be emphasized in Phase Four of your program.

There are certainly individuals who posses high levels of all three types of fitness, and we can "officially" call them fit. However, there are many people who have ignored all three areas of fitness and are, therefore, relatively *un*fit. But it is also possible to be relatively fit in one or two areas of fitness and still be unfit in one or two of the others. In fact, among many people who exercise, that's exactly the case. Typically, people do what's easiest for them or what they're already good at—and that's *all* they do. This means that they're ignoring the types of exercises that will do them the most amount of good. In fact, there's an old rule in the gym that states: "The exercise that you least enjoy is the one that will benefit you the most."

Each of the three areas of fitness represents an important piece in the overall fitness and weight loss puzzle, and you'll perform exercises that are specific to each of these three areas of fitness during the course of your program.

Get with the Program addresses each of these three areas of fitness just as it does everything else—progressively. This means that you will emphasize different elements of fitness when you are ready *and* when they will have the greatest overall positive effect for you.

While both your cardiovascular fitness and your muscular fitness have a greater overall effect on your metabolism, a sufficient level of functional fitness needs to be achieved *before* you can effectively train the other two areas. The exercises that you will be using to improve your functional fitness fall into four categories:

> flexibility exercises (stretches)
>
> abdominal crunches
>
> back and shoulder exercises
>
> lower leg exercise

In Phase One, the entire series of functional exercises can be completed in about eight to ten minutes. Go put on some comfortable clothing that is suitable for some light stretching and basic movement in order that you may practice these exercises *while* you read about them. *They should be performed at least three times a week, starting right now.*

Flexibility Exercises (Stretches)

Your flexibility refers to how well your joints and muscles move throughout a range of motion. Your flexibility decreases with age, particularly the flexibility of your joints. Your flexibility can also be diminished by inactivity or through excessive or improperly performed exercise.

It's no secret that flexibility exercises are frequently ignored when many people begin a structured fitness regimen, perhaps because stretching exercises take up additional time. (Of course, not having enough time is the most common excuse given for not doing any type of exercise.) But I assure you that the five flexibility exercises I will show you can be learned quickly and will be well worth the three to five minutes, three to five times a week, that they will require.

You should hold each stretch for five seconds, then relax it for five seconds. The stretch and release is performed at least three times (on each side of the body, if applicable). Do not bounce. Breathe deeply but comfortably during each stretch. Practice each one now as you read the descriptions, and check off each one when you've mastered the technique.

THE HAMSTRING STRETCH

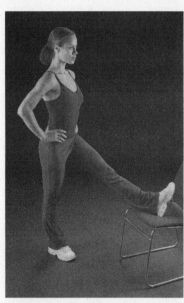

STARTING POSITION

While standing, place one foot on a chair, with the toes of that foot pointing up toward the ceiling. Keep both legs straight, with your knees locked but not hyperextended. With your hands on your hips, gradually bend forward until you feel a gentle tension in the back of the thigh (the hamstring) of the elevated leg. Hold this stretch for five seconds, then relax it for five seconds; hold it again for five seconds, then relax it for five seconds; hold it again for five seconds, then relax it for five seconds. Repeat this procedure on the opposite side. Be sure to breathe deeply but naturally during the entire stretch.

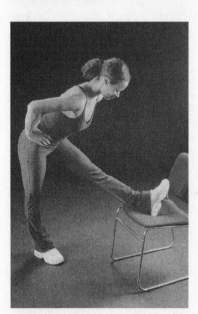

ACTIVE POSITION

QUADRICEPS STRETCH

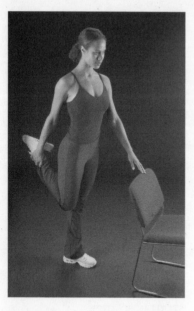

While using one hand to hold on to something, such as a chair, for support, use your other hand to grab your ankle and bend your leg, bringing your heel up toward your buttocks until you a feel gentle tension in the front of your thigh. The closer you can bring your heel to your buttocks, the more flexible you are. Your knee of the opposite leg should be slightly bent; keep your knees parallel. Hold this stretch for five seconds, then relax it for five seconds; hold it again for five seconds, then relax it for five seconds; hold it again for five seconds, then relax it for five seconds. Repeat this procedure on the opposite side. Be sure to breathe deeply but naturally during the entire stretch.

UPPER CALF STRETCH

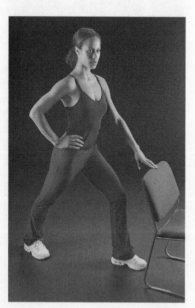

While using one hand to hold on to something, such as a chair, for support, place your other hand on your hip. Keep one leg straight out behind you, with your heel on the ground. Bend the opposite leg in front of you while keeping your knee directly over the corresponding foot (not ahead of it). The stretch should be felt in the upper calf of the leg that is straight back. If you don't feel it, bring the front leg (the one that's bent) farther forward. Again, you should feel a gentle tension. Do not arch your back. Hold this stretch for five seconds, then relax it for five seconds; hold it again for five seconds, then relax it for five seconds; hold it again for five seconds, then relax it for five seconds. Repeat this procedure on the opposite side. Be sure to breathe deeply but naturally during the entire stretch.

LOWER CALF STRETCH

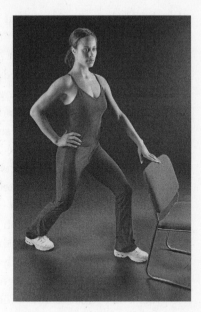

While using one hand to hold on to something, such as a chair, for support, place your other hand on your hip. Place one foot ahead of the other and bend your knees. Bring your hips slowly down toward the floor, keeping both heels on the ground. You should feel a gentle tension in the lower calf of your back leg. Do not arch your back. Hold this stretch for five seconds, then relax it for five seconds; hold it again for five seconds, then relax it for five seconds; hold it again for five seconds, then relax it for five seconds. Repeat this procedure on the opposite side. Be sure to breathe deeply but naturally during the entire stretch.

MIDDLE AND LOWER BACK STRETCH

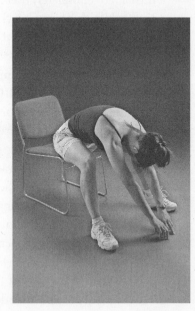

Sit on a chair with your knees apart and stretch out your arms in front of you. Gradually bend forward, keeping your arms stretched out and between your knees. Reach down toward the floor until you feel a gentle tension in your upper and/or middle back. Hold this stretch for five seconds, then relax it for five seconds; hold it again for five seconds, then relax it for five seconds; hold it again for five seconds, then relax it for five seconds. Be sure to breathe deeply but naturally during the entire stretch.

Abdominal Crunches

One of the most important muscle groups, and often the most over-looked, is the abdominal group. Anytime you lift something, even when you bend over to pick up a piece of paper, you need strong abdominal muscles to stabilize your body and protect your back. As you take on the challenges of exercise training, it's even more essential to take the time to strengthen this essential muscle group.

Before you practice these exercises, however, I first want to dispel a myth that never seems to die. Many people are under the false impression that doing abdominal exercises will reduce the amount of fat in the ab-dominal region. Unfortunately, there is no such thing as spot reducing—in *any* area of your body. But having a strong midsection does allow you to move faster and better, which in turn helps you to decrease the amount of body fat all over your body. Abdominal crunches can *indirectly* help you to reduce and control your body fat.

Since the abdomen is a group of muscles that act to stabilize and inte-grate other muscles and joints, it is best strengthened using a variety of specific exercises and body positions. I don't particularly care for the ab-dominal machines that have become so popular. For one thing, they make it difficult to completely exercise all of the muscles of the abdomen. In ad-dition, while these devices claim to protect your neck by resting it on a pad, what they do is prevent your neck from getting stronger and most people need to strengthen their necks. While it's true that the neck is slightly more vulnerable to injury during exercise, *not* to train it will insure that it will stay vulnerable! Crunches, when properly performed, train both your abdomen and your neck together.

Take note that the exercises shown below are crunches and not sit-ups. A number of years ago, sit-ups were used to strengthen the abdomen until it was discovered that the traditional sit-up places unnecessary stress on the back. By fully raising the torso, the hip flexor muscles can become tight, causing or exacerbating back problems. Crunches are similar, but the torso is raised only about thirty to forty-five degrees off the floor, and the knees are always bent (with the exception of the reverse trunk curl).

Now, let's take a look at the abdominal crunches. Keep in mind that these exercises are not intended for those with serious back problems. In addition, they may not be appropriate for individuals with neck condi-tions, heart problems, or high blood pressure. If any of the following exercises cause pain or discomfort other than that associated with normal muscular strengthening, discontinue their use and consult your physician. Practice these crunches now as you read the descriptions, and check off each one when you've mastered the technique.

Perform each of the four crunches shown below, fifteen times, at least three times a week, during Phase One.

THE BASIC CRUNCH

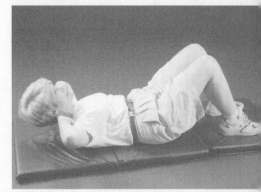

WITH NECK SUPPORTED, PHASES ONE AND TWO

Lie faceup on the floor. Bend your knees and place your heels twelve to fifteen inches from your buttocks. Place your hands lightly behind your neck. Use your abdominal muscles to raise your torso off the floor. Your chin should go straight up toward the ceiling with no flexion or rolling of your neck. Be sure to keep your shoulders square throughout the entire exercise. You should raise your torso up to a thirty- to forty-five-degree angle. Pause for a split second before returning to the starting position. Exhale on your way up and inhale upon returning to the starting position. Continue until the entire set of fifteen is complete. Once your neck is strengthened (typically within a month or two of performing these exercises), try resting your hands lightly on your collarbone while performing this exercise.

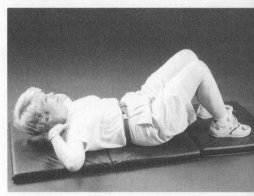

UNSUPPORTED, PHASES THREE AND FOUR

THE TWISTING TRUNK CURL CRUNCH

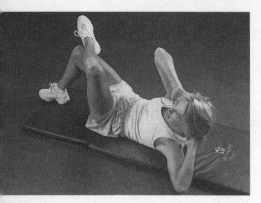

Lie faceup on the floor. Bend your knees and place your heels twelve to fifteen inches from your buttocks, as in the Basic Crunch. Place your left ankle on your right knee. Place your hands lightly behind your neck. Use your abdominal muscles to raise your left shoulder up toward your right knee; your shoulder should only be eight to twelve inches off the floor. Pause for a split second at the top and then return to the floor. Be sure to use your right arm, which is resting on the floor, as a fulcrum, or pivot point. Exhale on your way up and inhale upon returning to the starting position. Continue until the entire set of fifteen is complete. Take a deep breath and switch to the other side so that your right ankle is on your left knee, then repeat the process on this side.

THE UPPER ABDOMEN CRUNCH

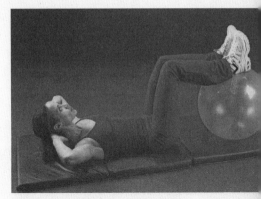

WITH NECK AND LEGS SUPPORTED, PHASES ONE AND TWO

Lie faceup on the floor. Raise your legs off the floor and bend them at a ninety-degree angle. It's a good idea to support your legs with a chair or exercise ball, or to place your feet on the wall until you are strong enough to hold them at a ninety-degree angle on your own. Place your hands lightly behind your neck. Use your abdominal muscles to raise your torso off the floor. Your chin should go straight up toward the ceiling with no flexion or rolling of the neck. Be sure to keep your shoulders square. Raise your torso up to a thirty- to forty-five-degree angle. Pause for a split second before returning to the starting position. Exhale on your way up and inhale upon returning to the starting position. Continue until the entire set of fifteen is complete. As your neck is strengthened, you may rest your hands lightly on your collarbone.

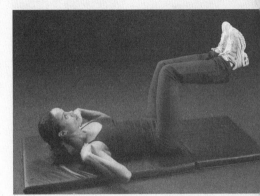

UNSUPPORTED, PHASES THREE AND FOUR

REVERSE TRUNK CURL

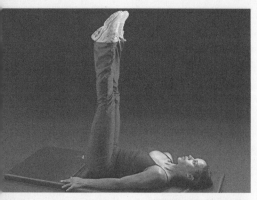

STARTING POSITION

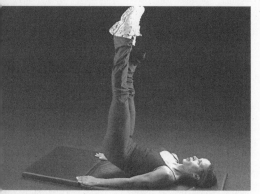

ACTIVE PHASE

This one takes some practice!

Lie faceup on the floor with your legs straight up, perpendicular to the ground. Keep your palms facedown and at your sides, and bend your knees slightly. Your entire back should remain flat on the floor, as should your shoulder blades. Contract your abdominal muscles, then curl your pelvis up, making your feet go up toward the ceiling. Begin to exhale upon contraction of your abdominal muscles. You should raise your hips only three to five inches off the floor. Be sure your legs and buttocks remain relaxed; the primary work should be done by your abdominal muscles. Pause for a split second before returning to the starting position. Exhale on your way up and inhale upon returning to the starting position. Continue until the entire set of fifteen is complete.

If you've never done these before, they may be difficult for you, and you may have to gradually build up to completing the entire set of fifteen.

Back and Shoulder Exercises

Along with the muscles of your abdomen, the muscles of your back have the important task of stabilizing your torso. Your back will especially benefit from the two exercises shown below. The Arm and Leg Raise strengthens the lower back, and the Shrug Roll strengthens the upper back. While all of the functional exercises you'll perform improve your posture, the Shrug Roll in particular is an excellent exercise for this because it strengthens your shoulders as well as your upper back. It should be performed without holding weights in Phases One and Two; for Phases Three and Four, you should hold a five- or ten-pound dumbbell while performing the exercise.

ARM AND LEG RAISE

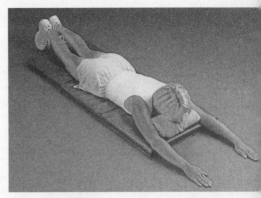

STARTING POSITION

You may have to build up to fifteen repetitions on this exercise!

Lie facedown on the floor with your head supported by a folded towel and your arms extended over your head. Contract your abdominal muscles and the muscles of your lower back. Raise your right arm and your left leg simultaneously. Keep your shoulders and your pelvis pressed against the floor. Do not lift your arm or leg too far; you should feel a gentle tension in your lower back muscles. Return your arm and leg to the floor. Exhale on your way up and inhale upon returning to the starting position. Continue until the entire set of fifteen is complete. Take a deep breath and begin on the other side, lifting your left arm and right leg.

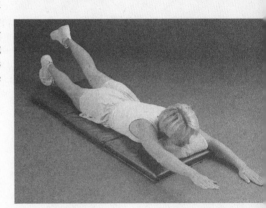

ACTIVE POSITION

THE SHRUG ROLL

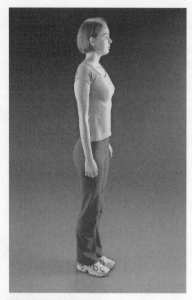

Stand erect with your feet shoulder-width apart. Keep your arms down at your sides. Begin the exercise by bringing your shoulders up toward your ears as high as your shoulders will go. Pause for a second at the top of this range of motion, then roll your shoulders back while squeezing your shoulder blades together. Again, pause for a second, then drop your shoulders back to the starting position. You should simply breathe naturally throughout this entire exercise. Continue until the entire set of fifteen is complete.

In Phases Three and Four, the amount of weight that you select for the Shrug Roll should not cause undue strain but should cause a slight burning sensation by about the tenth repetition. Since there is very little movement of the weight in this exercise, you can probably use more weight than you think you can. Begin with a five- or ten-pound dumbbell in each hand. If you can complete fifteen repetitions easily, you probably should add more weight.

**STARTING POSITION,
PHASES ONE AND TWO**

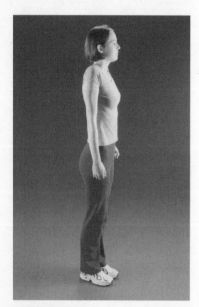

ACTIVE PHASE

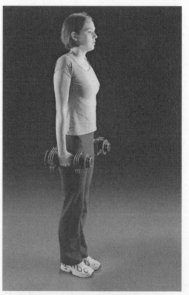

**PERFORMED WITH WEIGHTS,
PHASES THREE AND FOUR**

Lower Leg Exercise

The muscles of your calf and shin help you to stabilize your body when you stand and when you perform activities such as walking and climbing stairs. It's important to strengthen your lower legs so that your exercise becomes as effective as it can and because the shin is particularly vulnerable to an inflammatory condition known as shinsplints. You're particularly vulnerable to this condition when you walk, jog, or climb stairs, or when you begin an exercise program or increase the level of your current program. In fact, approximately 60 percent of those just beginning a walking program will experience some degree of shinsplints. In most cases, a program of stretching combined with strengthening exercises for the calf and shin as well as properly warming up will prevent this problem. The exercise I recommend for strengthening both your calves and your shins is the Heel Raise.

THE HEEL RAISE

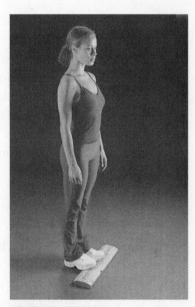

This exercise is best performed standing on a board approximately two inches by six inches by thirty-six inches or any raised, stable surface. Stand with the ball of each foot on the raised surface and with your heels on the floor. While keeping your feet approximately twelve inches apart and your knees straight but not hyperextended, slowly raise your heels as high as possible and hold for a split second before slowly returning to the starting position. You should exhale on your way up and inhale upon returning to the starting position. Continue until the entire set of fifteen is complete. In Phases Three and Four, you will perform this exercise holding dumbbells. Begin with a five- or ten-pound dumbbell in each hand. If you feel you can complete fifteen repetitions easily, you probably should add more weight.

STARTING POSITION

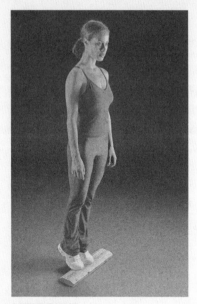

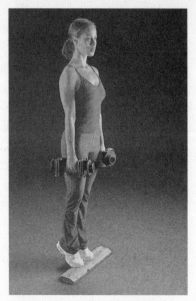

ACTIVE PHASE   **ACTIVE PHASE WITH DUMBBELLS**

These are the functional exercises that you will perform throughout your program. The stretches will remain the same throughout all of the phases. In Phase One, you will perform each of the functional exercises a total of fifteen times, three times a week. In Phase Two, you'll do one set of fifteen of each of the functional exercises, four times a week. In Phase Three you will do two sets of fifteen of each of the functional exercises, five times a week. In Phase Four, you'll do three sets of fifteen of each of the functional exercises, five times a week.

JUST A FEW LAST-MINUTE DETAILS

Following each phase in this book you will find your Get with the Program Journal. This is the basis for a complete record of your entire health and fitness journey and will help you organize everything that you will need to do along the way. Your journal will serve as a record of your progress, and it can be a great motivational tool. I highly recommend that you take the time to complete all of the journal entries. It's also a good idea to jot down your thoughts and feelings about this entire process, including what's easy for you, what's difficult, when you surprise yourself, and when you let yourself down. The information can prove to be invaluable. This permanent diary of your progress will also be fun and interesting to refer back to once you reach your goals.

Jennifer's Journal

I thought Jennifer, a client I worked with a number of years ago, would especially benefit from keeping a journal of her eating and exercise habits. She agreed. We also agreed that about once a month we would review any sections of her journal that she thought were appropriate for me to see. After the first month of working together, she told me that she didn't have anything to discuss. I asked again the next month, and she said that there was nothing to look at this time either. She was having such good results that I didn't feel the need to review her journal, but in the third month when she said there was nothing to review, I commented that she must really be on track. At that point she said, "No, not really. I've bought four journals to date, and each time I start to write in one, I'll have about six or seven good days, followed by a really bad eating day. After each bad day I throw the journal out and go buy another one and start all over." We both had a good laugh about that one, but the point of the story is that your journal is not simply a record of your good days. In fact, you'll discover more about yourself and benefit your program to a much greater extent by learning about your bad days. So include everything that you can think of that will benefit you and your program.

Get with the Program Journal—Phase One

By now you should have a good idea of what's expected of you in Phase One. If you're unclear or confused about any of the information discussed this far, please go back and reread it. Use the following checklist to make sure that by now you have:

❑ Read all of the information up through this section at least once and understand it.

❑ Contacted your physician and received clearance to participate in an exercise program.

❑ Started drinking your six glasses of water each day.

❑ Taken the twelve-question attitude quiz on page 19.

❑ Performed the written exercises corresponding to the questions that you answered yes to.

❑ Written the essay about any failed past attempts to lose weight.

❑ Signed the Get with the Program Contract with Myself (see page 53).

❑ Practiced and feel comfortable performing all of the functional exercises.

❑ Cleared time in your schedule to fulfill the requirements for this program.

❑ Informed those close to you that your goals and this program are important to you.

General Health Information

Starting weight _____ Blood pressure _____ Total cholesterol _____

LDL cholesterol _____ HDL cholesterol _____ Blood sugar _____

Phase One Requirements

Water: six glasses each day
Functional exercises: one set of fifteen, three times per week
Recommended time at Phase One: one to three weeks

PHASE ONE—WEEK ONE

	Water (8-ounce glasses)	Functional Exercises (1 set)	Comments About This Week
Monday			
Tuesday			
Wednesday			
Thursday			
Friday			
Saturday			
Sunday			
Weekly Totals			
Weekly Target	6	3	

PHASE ONE—WEEK TWO

Monday			
Tuesday			
Wednesday			
Thursday			
Friday			
Saturday			
Sunday			
Weekly Totals			
Weekly Target	6	3	

PHASE ONE—WEEK THREE

Monday			
Tuesday			
Wednesday			
Thursday			
Friday			
Saturday			
Sunday			
Weekly Totals			
Weekly Target	6	3	

If you can check off the following statements as being true . . .

❏ I fully understand all of the information contained in Phase One.
❏ I've completed at least one full week of drinking 6 eight-ounce glasses of water each day.
❏ I've completed my functional exercises three times a week for at least one week.
❏ I've looked at the requirements of Phase Two, and I'm confident I can meet the challenge.

. . . you're ready to move on to Phase Two. Congratulations!

REVVING UP YOUR METABOLISM

Congratulations on reaching Phase Two! In this phase you're going to start revving up your metabolism and getting in shape—slowly but surely—with the help of aerobic exercise. You're also going to limit the amount of alcohol that you consume, if that is one of your beverages of choice. These, as well as continuing to build on what you learned in Phase One, will be your primary goals in Phase Two.

You should be able to complete Phase Two in between three weeks and three months. Just remember that your progress should always be at your own pace. You might even be content with the results that you achieve here and decide that Phase Two is as far as you'd like to progress. That's fine. If you do, however, I would strongly recommend that you at least read the material about emotional eating in Phase Three.

In Phase One, you were drinking six glasses of water each day. I want you to add another glass, so you're now drinking seven glasses each day. And you will increase your functional exercises to four times a week instead of three. In Phase Two, you will be exercising aerobically a minimum of fifty minutes each week. Then, assuming that you want further results, you will progress to a goal of seventy-five minutes each week as you prepare for Phase Three. Finally, you're going to limit, or eliminate, your consumption of alcohol.

Goals for Phase Two

- Drink a minimum of seven glasses of water each day.
- Increase your functional exercise routine to four times per week.
- Perform aerobic exercise for a minimum of fifty minutes per week.
- Begin to limit, or eliminate, your consumption of alcohol.
- If you want to progress, increase your aerobic exercise to seventy-five minutes per week as you prepare for Phase Three.
- Maintain your exercise log.

ADDING AEROBIC EXERCISE TO YOUR LIFE

Aerobic exercise will soon become the foundation of your fitness routine. It is the primary way that you'll improve your cardiovascular (or aerobic) fitness, which in turn will increase your metabolism. Remember that cardiovascular fitness refers to the ability of your heart, lungs, and arteries to deliver oxygen (which is carried in the blood) to working muscles *and* your muscles' ability to use that oxygen to perform work over a particular period of time. By increasing your level of cardiovascular fitness, you are increasing the *rate* that your body can burn calories. I can't stress enough how important this is!

Increasing your cardiovascular fitness will have an immediate and significant impact on your metabolism and therefore your weight loss results. Increasing your metabolism is essential for creating the dramatic changes that will take place to your body. It will be a primary reason that you will maintain a lower percentage of body fat.

You'll also reap the benefits of a stronger heart, more powerful lungs, and more toned muscles.

Aerobic exercise should not be confused with strength training exercises. Aerobic exercise has a dulling effect on your appetite as opposed to strength training exercises, which will significantly *increase* your appetite. Strength training exercises are essential for your long-term health and weight management, so you'll be adding those exercises in Phase Four, at which time your eating choices will be better under control and your exercise habits firmly in place.

SELECTING AN AEROBIC EXERCISE

Aerobic exercises require you to use a lot of oxygen. When you train your body using a highly aerobic exercise, such as power walking or aerobic dancing, you are essentially raising the body's need to provide and utilize more oxygen. While you're exercising, your body's elevated need for oxygen triggers higher breathing rates and an increased heart rate. Consistently sending this same message through regular aerobic exercise—that you need additional oxygen—strengthens your heart and lungs (your cardiovascular system). But perhaps the most important information that this message sends is that you require a greater ability to utilize oxygen. This eventually leads your body to produce and store more of the aerobic enzymes that are found mostly within your muscles. More aerobic enzymes will help you burn more fat, so obviously you want a lot of them. And while the elevation in your heart rate and your breathing rate is immediate when you begin to exercise, the increase in the amount of aerobic enzymes occurs over a period of weeks and months. This is why it takes time before you're capable of increasing the amount of work you can perform during exercise. This is the essence of training. This process of training also works in reverse: When you are inactive, especially over a period of years, your muscles lose the ability to use oxygen and, therefore, lose the ability to burn calories. This is one of the reasons that your metabolism decreases over time, especially when you're inactive, and *why so many people regain their lost weight.*

In general, the more aerobic an exercise is, the greater effect it will have on your aerobic enzymes, cardiovascular fitness, and metabolism—and ultimately your percentage of body fat.

When you train your cardiovascular system using aerobic exercise, it's essential to:

1. Select primarily aerobic exercises to perform.

2. Perform your aerobic exercises continuously and for enough duration to get cardiovascular improvement.

3. Perform your aerobic exercises for enough total minutes each week to get cardiovascular improvement.

4. Perform your aerobic exercises at an intensity that improves your cardiovascular system.

5. Progress the amount of time you perform aerobic exercise each week to continue getting both cardiovascular improvement and weight loss results.

When training to improve your cardiovascular fitness, you want to select exercises that are *highly* aerobic, and there's no question that some exercises are more effective than others. In any given week, it's best to perform more than one type of aerobic exercise. This technique is called cross-training and leads to an overall higher level of fitness because a greater number of muscles become more highly trained at burning calories. You will also be less prone to overuse injuries when you vary the types of aerobic exercises that you perform. The most effective aerobic exercises are those that cause you to support all or most of your own body weight.

The Most Effective Aerobic Exercises

The "A" List

power walking

jogging

aerobic dancing

stair climbing

These four aerobic exercises represent the best choices to satisfy your weekly aerobic exercise program because they are not only highly aerobic but also relatively easy to build into your life.

The "B" List

stair stepping

elliptical exercise

Spinning

stationary cycling

indoor rowing

indoor cross-country skiing

These are exercises that, while not quite as aerobic as those in the "A" list, offer good alternatives.

The "C" List

jumping rope

in-line skating

outdoor cycling

outdoor rowing

outdoor cross-country skiing

These are exercises that aren't quite as effective as those in the first two lists. This may be due to the fact that they can be difficult to regularly build into your life, are too strenuous for you to perform for long enough to derive cardiovascular improvement, are dependent on the weather, or may require a specialized skill. However, if you are able to perform these exercises, they most definitely qualify toward your weekly aerobic minutes.

The "D" List

recumbent cycling

swimming

recreational sports

Finally, these are exercises that don't represent the best aerobic choices because their contribution to the weight loss process is minimal, but they can, on occasion, be used toward satisfying your weekly quota. *But you only get credit for half of the amount of time that you participate in these activities.* In other words, if you swim for twenty minutes, only ten minutes count toward your weekly aerobic minutes.

To help you choose which exercises are best for you, I've covered the pros and cons of each below. For each exercise I've included an aerobic rating, a convenience rating, a risk of injury rating, an overall rating, and comments regarding who this exercise is most appropriate for and who it's not appropriate for. All of the numbered ratings are from one to ten, ten being the best rating.

The "A" List

Power Walking

Aerobic rating: 7–8
Convenience rating: 10
Risk of injury rating: Low
Overall rating: 9
This exercise is appropriate for: Just about everyone.
This exercise is not appropriate for: Anyone with orthopedic complications that make walking impossible or difficult. Also, very fit individuals who would benefit from a more vigorous activity.

Power walking is my favorite overall aerobic exercise, and it's the one most people should start with. The chances of injuring yourself are quite low, it's extremely convenient, and it can be highly aerobic (but only when performed properly). The majority of my clients power walk for at least some of their weekly exercise.

If you want this exercise to count toward your weekly quota of exercise minutes, you'll want to be sure that you are power walking and not just walking. There is a distinct difference between the two. And if there is a downside to walking as a weight loss exercise, it's the fact that most people perform it at a very low intensity, much like they would walk to the store. In other words, they simply stay in their comfort zone.

To properly perform the technique of power walking, you need to use good posture: Keep your chin up and look straight out in front of you; be sure your shoulders are pulled up and back. Keep your arms bent at a ninety-degree angle and swing them with your fists coming up to shoulder level before swinging back down.

If you power walk consistently, your pace should get faster the more you do it. This is a sign your cardiovascular system is getting stronger and your metabolism is revving up. I'll tell you a secret: As your pace gets faster, your percentage of body fat is decreasing.

Power walking performed on a treadmill has the distinct advantage of allowing you to control the grade, or hill. It also allows you not to be dependent on the weather.

Practice your power walking now if you like. Once you're confident about your form, you can take a test walk and work on the pace that will bring you results. To help you determine what your appropriate pace is, refer to the section on intensity on page 108.

JOGGING

Aerobic rating: 10
Convenience rating: 10
Risk of injury rating: Moderate to high
Overall rating: 8
This exercise is appropriate for: Relatively fit individuals with no orthopedic or medical complications.
This exercise is not appropriate for: Beginning exercisers. Anyone with orthopedic complications that jogging would aggravate. Those whom a physician would not clear for vigorous exercise. This may include individuals with heart disease, lung disease, high cholesterol, high blood pressure, and/or smokers.

Jogging is a highly aerobic activity that can produce quick weight loss results. It's also quite convenient to perform. However, jogging is a high-impact exercise and carries the risk of a variety of overuse injuries. Jogging may not be your best choice if you have high blood pressure or heart problems, are quite overweight, smoke cigarettes, or have any other medical condition that would be aggravated with such a vigorous activity. Your physician can help you decide if jogging is right for you.

AEROBIC DANCING

Aerobic rating: 8
Convenience rating: 7
Risk of injury rating: Low for low-impact aerobics; moderate to high for high-impact aerobics
Overall rating: 7
This exercise is appropriate for: Individuals of all fitness levels. Those who enjoy rhythmic exercise as well as group exercise.

This exercise is not appropriate for: Anyone with orthopedic complications that aerobic dance movements would aggravate.

Aerobic dance can provide a fun way to accomplish your weekly exercise minutes. There is such a variety of classes these days that it's hard to get bored with this activity. Aerobic boxing and aerobic martial arts are considered to be in this category of exercise.

Keep in mind that there are high- and low-impact aerobics. I recommend the low-impact variety; you'll have much less risk of overuse and impact injuries. Luckily, these days most classes are the low-impact type. It's also best to attend a class taught by a knowledgeable instructor, preferably one certified by either the American Council on Exercise (ACE) or the Aerobics and Fitness Association of America (AFAA).

STAIR CLIMBING

Aerobic rating: 10
Convenience rating: 8
Risk of injury rating: Moderate
Overall rating: 8
This exercise is appropriate for: Those who can meet the strenuous demands of stair climbing. Those who have a limited amount of time to exercise and want a time-efficient, concentrated aerobic workout.
This exercise is not appropriate for: Anyone with orthopedic or medical complications that the intense nature of stair climbing would aggravate. This includes people with high blood pressure and smokers.

Stair climbing is actually a slightly different exercise than stair stepping, which will be covered on page 99. Stair climbing is performed on actual stairs, such as those that may be found in your home or at a stadium. Climbing actual stairs is fully weight supporting and is more aerobic than stair stepping on a machine. This is a great aerobic activity; however, you may have to build up to being able to perform it continuously for a minimum of 10 minutes. Simply walk up the stairs to the top, and then walk back down. Since going up is much more strenuous than going down, you should maintain the proper intensity by going down the stairs more quickly than you go up. Also, refer to the section on intensity on page 108 for guidelines about how hard you should work.

The "B" List

While slightly less aerobic than the preceding four exercises, the six exercises covered below are good alternatives and are especially appropriate for individuals with orthopedic and medical complications that prevent them from doing fully weight-bearing exercise.

STAIR STEPPING

Aerobic rating: 7
Convenience rating: 7
Risk of injury rating: Low
Overall rating: 8
This exercise is appropriate for: Most people, especially those who have a limited amount of time to exercise and want a time-efficient, concentrated aerobic workout.
This exercise is not appropriate for: Anyone with orthopedic or medical complications that stair stepping would aggravate.

This exercise requires the use of a stair-stepping machine. I like it because it is fairly aerobic, it's easy to learn, and it doesn't place much stress on your body.

If you perform stair stepping as an aerobic exercise, watch your posture: Be sure to keep your shoulders back, your arms slightly bent, and your hands in light contact with the machine (for balance, not to support your body weight).

ELLIPTICAL EXERCISE

Aerobic rating: 6–7
Convenience rating: 7
Risk of injury rating: Low
Overall rating: 7
This exercise is appropriate for: Beginning exercisers. Individuals who have a difficult time performing weight-bearing exercises. Anyone with orthopedic or medical complications that prevents them from doing other aerobic exercises such as power walking, jogging, aerobic dancing, or stair stepping.
This exercise is not appropriate for: Anyone with orthopedic or medical

complications that prevent them from performing the unique elliptical motion. Very fit individuals who would benefit from a more intense exercise.

Elliptical exercise is sort of a combination between jogging and stair stepping. It requires the use of a specialized exercise machine called (what else?) an elliptical exercise machine. When these machines first came out, the movement involved was more of a sliding motion, which did not provide for a very aerobic workout. Most of the newer models allow you to exercise your arms as well as your legs, and they tend to require that you lift your legs higher than the old machines. This motion more closely resembling jogging and is therefore more aerobic. I like these machines because they do not put much stress on muscles and joints.

SPINNING

Aerobic rating: 8
Convenience rating: 7
Risk of injury rating: Low
Overall rating: 7.5
This exercise is appropriate for: Individuals of all fitness levels. Those who for any reason have difficulty with fully weight-bearing exercises.
This exercise is not appropriate for: Individuals prone to orthopedic complications, such as tendonitis that especially affects the knee, ankle, and/or hip. Also, those with certain types of back and/or neck conditions.

Spinning is a fitness trend that gained popularity in the midnineties and continues to be a force in the fitness industry. Spinning uses a specialized stationary bicycle, music, and an instructor who conducts the class. The instructor takes you on a cycling "journey" that involves a variety of intensities and body positions on the bike.

Spinning can be an exciting way to work out in a group setting. You don't have to learn a bunch of intricate moves or steps like in an aerobic dance class. And the music gets you moving!

The ability to add resistance to the wheel of the bike overcomes the fact that your weight is fully supported by the bike. All in all, Spinning is a good way to improve your cardiovascular fitness.

Be aware that the standard Spinning class lasts between fifty and ninety minutes, and that includes your warm-up and cooldown. Those of you that are in the beginning phases of the program may not be able to finish the entire class. That's fine. You only need to satisfy the requirements of your phase. Remember that within the average Spinning class you are exercising at the proper intensity for a total of thirty to forty minutes.

STATIONARY CYCLING

Aerobic rating: 6
Convenience rating: 8
Risk of injury rating: Low
Overall rating: 6
This exercise is appropriate for: Individuals of all fitness levels. Those who for any reason have difficulty with fully weight-bearing exercises.
This exercise is not appropriate for: Individuals prone to orthopedic complications, such as tendonitis that especially affects the knee, ankle, and/or hip. Also, those with certain types of back and/or neck conditions.

With stationary cycling, you typically don't work as hard as you would in a Spinning class. This is because you don't have an instructor pushing you and taking you through movements that require you to move up and down from your seat. However, this can be a rather convenient indoor exercise and a good way to get in your weekly minutes of aerobic exercise. Just be sure you maintain the proper intensity with this exercise.

INDOOR ROWING

Aerobic rating: 7
Convenience rating: 7
Risk of injury rating: Low
Overall rating: 7
This exercise is appropriate for: Individuals of all fitness levels. Those who for any reason have difficulty with fully weight-bearing exercises.
This exercise is not appropriate for: Individuals with certain back or neck conditions. Also, those prone to orthopedic complications that affect the hip, knees, ankles, shoulders, and/or elbows.

Indoor rowing is a fairly aerobic exercise that's quite easy to learn. It requires the use of a rowing machine. I like it mainly because it trains both your arms and legs. Just be sure not to hyperextend your back while rowing. This exercise is meant to be performed using 80 percent contribution from your legs and only 20 percent from your arms.

INDOOR CROSS-COUNTRY SKIING

Aerobic rating: 6.5
Convenience rating: 7
Risk of injury rating: Low
Overall rating: 6.5
This exercise is appropriate for: Individuals who are proficient at the cross-country skiing technique. Individuals of higher fitness levels.
This exercise is not appropriate for: Beginning exercisers. Anyone who is not proficient in the technique of cross-country skiing.

Indoor cross-country skiing is an aerobic activity that trains both your arms and legs. It requires the use of an indoor ski trainer. This is a good overall exercise once you learn the specialized technique.

The "C" List

JUMPING ROPE

Aerobic rating: 10 (if your good!)
Convenience rating: 9
Risk of injury rating: High
Overall rating: 7
This exercise is appropriate for: Relatively fit individuals. Those who possess rope-jumping skills.
This exercise is not appropriate for: Beginning exercisers. Anyone with orthopedic complications that heavy jumping would aggravate. Those for whom a physician would not clear for vigorous exercise. This may include individuals with heart disease, lung disease, high blood pressure, and/or smokers.

Jumping rope is a highly aerobic exercise, but only if you are good enough to maintain a continuous workout. Jumping rope is also tough on your body, leading to a variety of overuse injuries if it's done too often. But you can't beat the convenience, especially for traveling. All in all, I think jumping rope is best as an occasional activity, unless you can do it well and are relatively fit.

IN-LINE SKATING

Aerobic rating: 8 (if you're good!)
Convenience rating: 6

Risk of injury rating: High
Overall rating: 7
This exercise is appropriate for: Those who live in a region with weather conducive to consistently exercising outdoors. Those possessing the skills to perform in-line skating. Relatively fit individuals.
This exercise is not appropriate for: Individuals prone to orthopedic complications, such as tendonitis that especially affects the knee, ankle, and/or hip. Those with certain types of back and/or neck conditions. Those who are prone to accidents.

In-line skating is a moderately aerobic activity, but only if performed continuously. There are a few things to keep in mind if you're considering it as a regular activity. For one thing, in-line skating has a high injury rate from accidents. Don't forget to wear your helmet, knee pads, elbow pads, and wrist guards! It's important to find an area that has a minimum of traffic without a lot of stop signs or traffic lights. A paved area closed to automobile traffic is perfect.

And, of course, you're at the mercy of the weather.

Outdoor Cycling

Aerobic rating: 8
Convenience rating: 6
Risk of injury rating: Moderate to high
Overall rating: 6
This exercise is appropriate for: Those who live in a region with weather conducive to consistently exercising outdoors.
This exercise is not appropriate for: Individuals prone to orthopedic complications, such as tendonitis that especially affects the knee, ankle, and/or hip. Those with certain types of back and/or neck conditions. Those who are prone to accidents.

Outdoor cycling is a great way to log your weekly aerobic minutes. But if you do it, be sure to wear a helmet; accident rates from bicycling are high. And it's a good idea to select a route that has minimum traffic and few stoplights.

Outdoor Rowing

Aerobic rating: 6–8 (depending on the vessel)
Convenience rating: 5

Risk of injury rating: Low
Overall rating: 6
This exercise is appropriate for: Individuals of all fitness levels. Those who for any reason have difficulty with fully weight-bearing exercises.
This exercise is not appropriate for: Individuals with back or neck conditions. Also, those prone to orthopedic complications that affect the hip, knees, ankles, shoulders, and/or elbows.

This requires access to a body of water and a vessel. A rowing scull is the most aerobic vessel to row in due to the heavy contribution of both arms and legs. A kayak is somewhat less aerobic than using a scull, but it still provides a good aerobic workout. With a canoe, you are using primarily your arms; this vessel therefore does not represent the best choice. Regardless, outdoor rowing can be a fun way to accomplish your aerobic minutes. Not only do you get to enjoy the great outdoors, rowing doesn't place a great deal of stress on your body.

OUTDOOR CROSS-COUNTRY SKIING

Aerobic rating: 10
Convenience rating: 5
Risk of injury rating: Moderate
Overall rating: 7
This exercise is appropriate for: Individuals who live in a region with a climate conducive to skiing. Individuals who are proficient at the cross-country skiing technique. Very fit individuals.
This exercise is not appropriate for: Beginning exercisers. Anyone not proficient in the technique of cross-country skiing. Those prone to orthopedic complications that affect the hips, knees, ankles, shoulders, and/or elbows.

Outdoor cross-country skiing is considered the most aerobic all-around exercise. It thoroughly trains both your arms and legs. But, obviously, to perform this exercise, you need to live where there's snow. In addition, it requires a specialized technique that takes time to learn. Finally, you need to be rather fit to enjoy this vigorous activity.

The Fun But Not Optimal List

Remember that for the following activities you can only count half the number of minutes that you actually perform them.

RECUMBENT CYCLING

Aerobic rating: 5
Convenience rating: 7
Risk of injury rating: Low
Overall rating: 6
This exercise is appropriate for: Those who are not overly concerned with losing weight. Anyone with orthopedic complications that prevent them from doing any other exercises.
This exercise is not appropriate for: Individuals whose primary goal is to lose weight. Very fit individuals.

Recumbent cycling requires the use of a recumbent bicycle. You are essentially bicycling while seated, with your legs out in front of you. Not only is all of your weight supported, but this exercise can be performed with little effort, which is why it is not highly recommended as a weight loss exercise. However, it is appropriate while recovering from an injury or as an occasional break. It's also a great warm-up!

SWIMMING

Aerobic rating: 7
Convenience rating: 6
Risk of injury rating: Low
Overall rating: 6
This exercise is appropriate for: Those who are not overly concerned with losing weight. Anyone with orthopedic complications that prevent them from doing any other exercises. Very fit individuals who are skilled swimmers.
This exercise is not appropriate for: Individuals whose primary goal is to lose weight. And nonswimmers!

I wouldn't recommend that you use swimming as your main source of aerobic exercise. Swimming used to be one of the most prescribed exercises for weight loss. This would seem reasonable because swimming is fairly aerobic and it doesn't place a lot of stress on your body, which is especially important if you're carrying a lot of weight. The problem with swimming is that it doesn't allow your body to heat up, which is one of the benefits of other aerobic exercises. The exercise of swimming, combined with the cooling effect of the water, increases your appetite. In addition, if you are carrying a lot of fat weight, you're going to be more buoyant and therefore your body is not going to work as hard as that of a leaner individual. These things make swimming one of the least effective weight loss exercises.

Recreational Sports

When you participate in recreational sports such as tennis, basketball, and volleyball, the aerobic training is intermittent. But take heart, you can still use half of the minutes that you play these activities. And they do tend to add a little variety to your workouts.

HOW LONG SHOULD YOU CONTINUOUSLY EXERCISE?

I've heard many theories through the years about how long you should continuously exercise to maximize the weight loss benefit of exercise. Many of those theories are based on the fact that when you first start exercising, you burn mostly carbohydrates that are stored within your muscles and organs. After a few minutes, you start to burn increasingly higher percentages of stored fat. For years, this knowledge led many exercise professionals to prescribe long continuous bouts of rather low-intensity exercise for individuals who wanted to lose weight. It would seem to make sense that the longer you exercised, the higher percentage of fat you would burn and the more body fat you'd lose. But as it turns out, exercising continuously for long periods of time isn't as relevant to your weight loss efforts as once thought. You see, if you had to rely on the measly amount of fat that you burn during your exercise, you'd need three lifetimes to reach your goal. While this amount of fat loss does help the overall process a little, the *real* fat loss comes from your changed metabolism and your elevated amount of fat burning for twenty-four hours of each day of your life. In order for exercise to make the necessary increases to your metabolism, such as increasing your aerobic enzymes, it needs to be performed continuously for about ten minutes. (Fifteen minutes would be even better, but I'll take ten!) This provides the necessary stimulus for your cells to say, "Hey, we need to make some changes!" You will not count any exercise that is not continuously performed for at least ten minutes. If you go longer, then great; but ten minutes is the bare minimum.

HOW MUCH AEROBIC EXERCISE IS ENOUGH?

When it comes to your weight loss, the more aerobic exercise you perform (within reason!) the better. But let's get real! I know you have only so much time to devote to your exercise routine. How much time you do take will be strictly up to you. You'll have to consider several factors, such as the amount of time that you have available, medical concerns, and even your unique set of genetics and how they affect your results.

Research studies on exercise can give you some guidelines. As a general rule of thumb, if all you want to do is keep your heart, lungs, and circulatory system healthy, about thirty to forty minutes a week is adequate. If weight loss is your primary goal, a minimum of fifty minutes a week is recommended. And while some people will reach their weight loss goals by exercising fifty minutes a week, others will need more time to show significant success.

In Phase Two, you'll be aerobically exercising a minimum of fifty minutes a week. If you can do more, great. These fifty minutes should be spread throughout the week, meaning you should exercise on at least three different days and never allow more than two days to pass without getting some exercise in any given week. Finally, remember that you must exercise for *at least* ten minutes continuously for the time to count toward your weekly quota.

Your weekly aerobic minutes will be a key factor in your weight loss results. When you reach a real plateau in your results, simply increase the amount of weekly aerobic minutes that you perform or, if you're ready, move on to the next phase, or do both. One of your goals in Phase Two is to progress your weekly aerobic minutes to seventy-five, assuming you want further results and you plan on moving to Phase Three.

Before your aerobic minutes can have their full effect on your metabolism, however, you must control the most important factor regarding your aerobic exercise. Read on!

HOW HARD SHOULD YOU EXERCISE?

It's extremely important that you completely understand the information in this section. It includes one of the most important skills that you will need to learn. Without a doubt, how hard you work (the intensity of your exercise) is the most important component of your aerobic workout and one of the most important aspects of your entire weight loss process. The bottom line is that the more aerobic work you are able to perform within a given amount of time, the better cardiovascular shape you'll be in. And the better cardiovascular shape you're in, the lower the amount of body fat that you will maintain. In other words, I want you to exercise at the highest intensity that is safe for you *and* that you can maintain for your entire workout.

When I speak of working hard or working at a relatively high intensity, I'm speaking about the effort of which you are capable. This may be contrary to what you've done or been told in the past. You've probably heard that in order to burn fat, you must exercise for a long period of time at a slow pace. This is because a number of years ago several scientific studies showed that when a person exercised at a lower intensity level (below 70 percent of his maximum ability), he burned a higher percentage of stored fat (body fat) versus stored carbohydrates (glycogen). These studies also showed that as a person increased the intensity (or pace) of his workout, he began to burn a higher percentage of stored carbohydrates as opposed to stored fat. Since it's fat you want to get rid of, it might seem that the best way to accomplish that would be to slow down the intensity of your exercise to below 70 percent of your maximum ability—but it simply doesn't work that way.

Whether you're burning stored carbohydrates or stored fat during your workout doesn't matter much at all. What does matter is challenging your body's aerobic (or cardiovascular) power during your exercise sessions with moderately high-intensity exercise. Over time this causes an increase in your body's ability to provide oxygen to the muscles and an increase in your muscles' ability to utilize that oxygen. In short, your metabolism is increased, not simply during the time in which you're exercising, but 24 hours each day, 365 days a year! So don't get hung up on how many calories you burn during your exercise session. What is important is the *rate* that you're burning calories both during your exercise session—as well as the other 23½ hours of every day of your life. *That's* what produces dramatic results!

The truth, though, is that most of us feel much more comfortable with low-intensity exercise. In fact, when most people are left to their own devices, they will adopt an exercise intensity that is too low. This is a common reason why so many people give up soon after beginning an exercise program—they simply don't get the results they need in order to stay motivated.

I'll say it again:
Low-intensity exercise is not all that effective
in changing your metabolism!

In addition, when you exercise at a low intensity for long periods of time, you simply burn lots of calories, get very hungry, and eventually eat back all of the burned-off calories.

Remember:
The entire premise behind training is to challenge your
body and have it respond by getting stronger. Don't
challenge it and risk having little or no change take place.

With low-intensity exercise, you're barely challenging the cardiovascular system and doing little to improve your current level of fitness. Moderately high-intensity exercise increases your cardiovascular power, which increases your body's ability to perform work and leads to a higher metabolism. This decreases your set point and the amount of body fat that you'll maintain. In short, you get in better shape.

So don't be fooled: Calories burned during your workout aren't what is really important. Challenging your cardiovascular system is. You do this by exercising in "the zone."

What Exactly *Is* the Zone?

The zone is the intensity of exercise that safely produces the results that you want. If you exercise below the zone, you risk not getting results. If you exercise above the zone, you risk not being able to continue your exercise or, worse, you risk injury. The zone is the perfect intensity level at which to perform your cardiovascular exercise—between 70 and 80 percent of your maximum ability.

How do you know when you're in the zone? There are essentially two ways: taking your heart rate and monitoring your level of perceived exertion. Either way is acceptable, but for most people I prefer monitoring their level of perceived exertion.

Monitoring your heart rate during exercise is the most common way to tell you if you're in the zone. If you've ever taken an aerobics class or had someone give you an exercise prescription, you're probably familiar with the phrase "target heart rate range." But if you're not, it's a recommended range of heart rates (in beats per minute) that you should achieve during your exercise in order to safely train your cardiovascular system. It's derived by first obtaining your maximum heart rate. This can be measured directly by taking a maximum treadmill test (which must be administered by a health care professional) or estimated by subtracting your age from 220. To figure out your target heart rate, multiply your maximum heart rate by 80 percent. To estimate your target heart range, you add 5 (beats) to your target heart rate and subtract 5 (beats) from your target heart rate. The following example of this formula is for a forty-year-old individual.

Estimated maximum heart rate: $\qquad$ *220 − 40* $\qquad$ *= 180 beats per minute*
Target heart rate: $\qquad$ *180 × .80* $\qquad$ *= 144 beats per minute*
Target heart rate range: *[(144 − 5 = 139) and (144 + 5 = 149)] = 139 to 149 beats per minute*

The entire premise for using your heart rate to monitor the intensity of your aerobic exercise is based on the assumption that your heart rate accurately reflects your oxygen consumption, or how hard you're working aerobically. But there are a number of shortcomings in using your heart rate to monitor your exercise intensity. First, your heart rate doesn't always directly reflect how hard you're working or your oxygen consumption. There are a number of factors that can throw this relationship off, such as your emotional state, what you're thinking, medications you are taking, the temperature and the altitude you are in, and your caffeine consumption, to name a few. This could mean that although you're exercising at your prescribed target heart rate, you may be either working too hard or not hard enough due to a number of factors beyond your control. Second, the formula of 220 minus your age is only an estimation of your heart rate and is accurate for only about a third of the population. Third, to obtain an accurate maximum heart rate requires a maximum treadmill test. Most people do not want to incur the cost and inconvenience of having this test. Finally, have you ever taken your heart rate during exercise? Even if you're one of the lucky people whose target heart rate can be accurately calculated by the formula, trying to measure it during your workout can be next to impossible. You have to stop exercising, find your pulse, and count the number of heartbeats all in a matter of seconds so that your heart rate doesn't slow down too much. There are many people who couldn't find their pulse even if they were given an hour to do it!

Have you ever seen an athlete stop to check her pulse during a workout? Probably not! Athletes are simply in tune with their bodies. They instinctively know how hard they're working, and they adjust their exercise efforts based on a general feeling of fatigue and shortness of breath. There's no reason why you can't do the same. I teach this method of perceived exertion to all my clients on the first day we work together, and it works really well for most of them. It may take you one or two exercise sessions to get the hang of it, but it's well worth the effort.

If you're accustomed to using your target heart rate to monitor your exercise and you're comfortable using this method, by all means continue to do so. Also, if you have any medical condition that would be aggravated if you went above a certain heart rate, you'll need to keep track of exactly what your heart rate is when you exercise. Your physician can prescribe a training heart rate for you, and you may want to use a heart rate monitor to assure that you don't exceed your limit. But for most people, I prefer perceived exertion, a method that requires you to pay close attention to your body and what's happening to it. Perceived exertion is a subjective rating of how hard you're working during exercise that is based primarily on your breathing. Your breathing becomes elevated in direct response to your oxygen requirements and gives you immediate feedback about the intensity of your exercise. In addition, you don't have to stop exercising to "take a reading." You simply evaluate—using a scale from zero to ten— how hard you're working based primarily on how short of breath you are. Your optimum zone is anywhere between a rating of seven and eight. I want you to exercise *consistently* at level seven when you first start out.

Later you can stay at seven or move up to working at level eight, if and when you're ready.

Now let's take a look at the scale. Be sure to fully understand how you should feel at levels seven and eight, which is where you'll be exercising most of the time. Begin by picturing a scale from zero to ten.

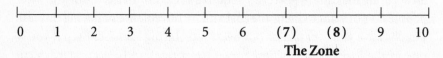

| 0 | 1 | 2 | 3 | 4 | 5 | 6 | (7) | (8) | 9 | 10 |

The Zone

What you should be feeling at each level:

0—This is the feeling you would experience at rest. There is no feeling of fatigue. Your breathing is not at all elevated. You will not experience this level during exercise.

1—This is the feeling you would experience while working at your desk or reading. There is no feeling of fatigue. Your breathing is not elevated.

2—This is the feeling you would experience while getting dressed. There is little or no feeling of fatigue. Your breathing is not elevated. You will rarely experience this low level during exercise.

3—This is the feeling you would experience while slowly walking across the room to turn on the television. There is little feeling of fatigue. You may be slightly aware of your breathing, but it is slow and natural. You may experience this right in the beginning of an exercise session.

4—This is the feeling you would experience while slowly walking outside. There is a very slight feeling of fatigue. Your breathing is slightly elevated, but comfortable. There is a slight feeling of fatigue. You should experience this level during the initial stages of your warm-up.

5—This is the feeling you would experience while walking to the store. There is a slight feeling of fatigue. You are aware of your breathing, which is deeper than that of level four. You should experience this level at the end of your warm-up.

6—This is the feeling you would experience when you are walking somewhere and are very late for an appointment. There is a general feeling of fatigue, but you know that you can maintain this level of exertion. Your breathing is deep and you are aware of it. You should experience this level in the transition from your warm-up to your exercise session and during the initial phase of learning how to work at level seven or eight.

7—This is the feeling you would experience when you are exercising vigorously. There is a definite feeling of fatigue, but you are quite sure you can maintain this level for the rest of your exercise session. Your breathing is deep and you are definitely aware of it. You could carry on a conversation, but you would probably choose not to do so. *This is the baseline level of exercise that you should maintain in your workout sessions.*

8—This is the feeling you would experience when you are exercising very vigorously. There is a definite feeling of fatigue, and if you asked yourself if you could continue for the remainder of your exercise session, your answer would be that you think you could, but you're not 100 percent sure. Your breathing is very deep. You could still carry on a conversation, but you don't feel like it. This becomes the feeling you should experience only after you are comfortable reaching level seven and are ready for a more intense workout. This is the level that produces rapid results for many people.

9—This is the feeling that you would experience if you were exercising very, very vigorously. You would experience a definite feeling of fatigue, and if you asked yourself if you could continue this pace for the remainder of your exercise session, your answer would be you probably could not. Your breathing is very labored. It would be very difficult to carry on a conversation. This is a feeling you may experience for short periods when trying to zero in on a level eight. This is a level that many athletes train at, and it is difficult for them. You should not be experiencing level nine on a routine basis and should slow up when you do.

10—You should not experience level ten. This is the feeling you would experience with all-out exercise. This level cannot be maintained for very long, and there is no benefit in reaching it.

Take the time to learn each level. Remember that you're striving to reach and maintain *level seven* when you first begin exercising. Later, once you are more highly trained, you can reach level eight during part or all of your exercise session.

Why Should You Exercise at a Level Seven or Eight?

Whether you use the target heart rate method or the rate of perceived exertion to monitor your exercise intensity, what you are really attempting to do is to exercise consistently at a certain percentage of your maximum ability. For example, if I asked you to do an all-out sprint, you would quickly reach 100 percent of your maximum ability to exercise (or what's known as your maximum oxygen consumption). You cannot maintain 100 percent of your maximum oxygen consumption for very long, and you wouldn't want to try; your workout will *always* be a percentage of this maximum ability. A ten on the perceived exertion scale corresponds to this level of 100 percent of your maximum oxygen consumption. A seven represents 70 percent of your maximum. An eight represents 80 percent. As long as you rate your exercise at seven or eight, you're in the zone!

Keep in mind that when you first exercise at level seven, you may not like the feeling, though you will get used to it. If you can't keep up the exertion of level seven at first, start at level six and then increase to level seven for one or two minutes at a time. Keep extending the amount of time that you do this until you are consistently working at level seven. Usually within a week or two after beginning, every client I've worked with has been able to exercise at level seven for at least ten or fifteen minutes.

You may have already figured out that the amount of work that you achieve at level seven will be different from your friend's or spouse's level seven. Level seven is relative to *you*. This is especially important to keep in mind if you exercise with someone else or in a group. Each person needs to stay within his own zone. That means, for example, if you're walking or jogging outside with a group, it may not be in the best interest of everyone to stay together for the workout. The common temptation is to work out together at the same rate, but don't give in. You can socialize after your workout is finished.

Suzanne's Story

I started working with Suzanne a couple of years ago. During her initial consultation, she had mentioned that she'd been power walking for over two years and that when she first started, she lost about ten pounds and had not lost a pound since. Her goal was to lose an additional twenty-five pounds. On her very first workout, I let her set the pace. There was no question that Suzanne had adopted a pace that was too comfortable for her and that this was the cause of her not showing results. While she walked, I could hear no elevation in her rate of breathing. In fact, there wasn't much difference between the way she was breathing while walking and while we were sitting and talking about her exercise.

We picked up the pace, and her breathing immediately became deeper and more frequent. I asked her if she could maintain this pace and she answered, "Yes!" We walked at that pace for thirty minutes. I told her that this was the pace at which she needed to exercise in order to get results. She then replied, "That was really challenging, but right now I feel exhilarated!" From that day on, Suzanne methodically lost two pounds a week.

Suzanne moved past her level of comfort—that's what you need to do, too. Realize that as your body becomes more highly trained, you will learn that the amount of exercise you can accomplish at level seven will increase. This is all part of the process of improving your level of fitness. What do you do, though, if your exercise starts to feel too easy for you and you notice that you're no longer getting results? This is when you pick up your pace!

HOW SHOULD YOU STEP UP YOUR AEROBIC EXERCISE PROGRAM?

I urge you not to make the mistake that many people do, which is to believe that once they have their routine down, all they need to do is show up and punch the exercise time clock. Exercise needs to be increased in duration and intensity if results are going to continue. In that way, you not only accomplish more work and become stronger, you also adjust your goals and set new ones for yourself. *Your progress helps you define where you want to go and how quickly you want to get there.* But before you decide how aggressively to move through the four phases of Get with the Program, I want you to fully understand how your body changes and your fitness improves.

Once you begin aerobic training on a regular basis, you will begin to experience improvements rather quickly in the amount of work you can perform and in your cardiovascular function. Why? Let's take a look at your first workout. In it, you'll be performing your exercise at a level above what your body routinely experiences in the normal course of a day. Let's say that you're power walking at level seven. Your muscles, primarily your leg muscles, will need even more oxygen than normal to perform this new level of exertion, so the muscles involved will send out signals to your brain that they need more oxygen sent to those working muscles. Your brain then sends a message to your lungs to breathe harder, putting more oxygen in the blood, and to your heart to beat faster, to move more blood. Since you're functioning at a higher aerobic level than your body normally is accustomed to, the working muscles probably don't have an adequate amount of aerobic enzymes to process all this additional oxygen; so to continue walking at level seven, you must provide energy anaerobically, or without oxygen, using a series of complex chemical reactions that occur within your muscles. The reactions lead to the production of lactic acid, which in turn makes you want to slow down or stop exercising. It also makes you sore in a day or two. The bottom line is that you didn't have enough aerobic enzymes to adequately perform the exercise at the level that you were pushing yourself at. In addition, your heart and lungs were not strong enough to deliver an ample supply of blood to the muscles. Is this a problem?

No. This is exactly what happens whenever you are trying to reach a higher level of fitness. This is what training is all about. What you are doing during an aerobic workout is modestly starving your body for oxygen. This sends the message to your heart that it must become stronger (just as the other muscles in your body become stronger when you train with weights), the message to your lungs that they must get stronger, and the message to your muscles that they need to manufacture more aerobic enzymes so that they can process more oxygen.

Your body responds by strengthening all of these systems. But these results are contingent upon depriving (only slightly) the body of oxygen while exercising. To continue to improve, you must continue to aerobically challenge your body on a regular basis! I'm not saying that you need to do something outside of your capabilities, but just to test your capabilities. This is why if you walk the same three miles at the same pace for three days a week, your cardiovascular health will eventually plateau, as will your overall fitness level and your weight.

Keep in mind that all of these changes take time to occur. The amount of time differs depending on the individual, but they always occur. You simply must be patient and persistent. *And be willing to improve.* Your progression is built into each phase of Get with the Program. But it's up to you to move yourself through those phases within your own time frame.

Now that you know all that you need to know about aerobic exercise, I want you to learn the importance of limiting your consumption of alcohol—the second goal of Phase Two.

LIMITING YOUR CONSUMPTION OF ALCOHOL

If you don't currently consume alcohol and don't plan to, you can skip this section. If you do imbibe, take the time to read this information and make your own decisions. I realize that drinking alcohol is a personal choice, and I'm not about to lecture you or say that you must give it up. But I *am* going to make a strong argument that you should attempt to limit your consumption of alcohol as much as possible. This will greatly improve your ability to reach a higher level of fitness and your goal weight.

Consuming alcohol has a few strikes against it when it comes to your body weight and your well-being. Alcohol's first problem is that it has a lot of calories! Take a look at the following comparison of calorie sources:

Carbohydrates = 4 calories per gram

Protein = 4 calories per gram

Alcohol = 7 calories per gram

Fat = 9 calories per gram

As you can see, alcohol has almost as many calories as pure fat, and when it comes to gaining weight, alcohol is even worse than eating pure fat. Fat has nutrients that you need, alcohol doesn't. Fat also plays a role in telling you when you're full, and the inclusion of it in your diet can actually help you stop eating at meals. Alcohol, however, is absorbed almost immediately from the stomach and dumped right into the bloodstream. From there, it can be quickly converted to body fat. Since it doesn't occupy any space in your stomach, you can drink it and then immediately fill up on foods to double the damage! But probably the worst effect of alcohol as far as your weight is concerned is that it slows down your metabolism. This effect can linger for days, changing the *rate* at which you burn calories. If that's not bad enough, alcohol consumption can have negative motivational effects as well. It's no secret that alcohol tends to dampen your enthusiasm for eating the right foods. And it certainly doesn't make you feel like having strong workouts. All told, alcohol derails your weight loss efforts in direct proportion to how much you consume. So my advice? Eliminate it if you can. If you're not willing to go that far, then at least cut your consumption in half. Simply estimate the amount of alcohol that you consume in an average week and cut that amount in half. This will dramatically help your weight loss efforts. I've found that even the most diehard connoisseurs have been able to successfully cut alcohol consumption in half and still appreciate the drinks they do have—maybe even to a greater extent. Isn't it really the first glass of wine that tastes the best anyway? Just stop to ask yourself after the first drink if subsequent drinks are really worth the damage.

Invariably someone asks me about studies that claim one or two glasses of wine a day is actually good for your health, particularly your heart. You also may have heard that a couple glasses of wine a day can lower your cholesterol. This is still being debated, and in fact, there are studies supporting both sides of the argument. One thing you should know is that a lot of these studies were done on a fairly sedentary population. These individuals are at much higher risk for heart disease and cholesterol problems than an active person. The main point is that a program of eating right, exercising regularly, and limiting excessive consumption of alcohol would have a much greater positive effect on your heart and your health than the vague and generic advice of having a drink or two each day. Granted there are individuals who may benefit from the blood-thinning effects of alcohol, and their physicians may even recommend moderate consumption. But even if alcohol is beneficial for certain people, no one should use this as a license to overindulge. What is certain is that *too much* alcohol is bad for your heart, liver, and various other parts of your body on top of contributing to weight problems. So make your plan now to cut down and start reaping the rewards.

Beth's Story

Beth wanted to lose ten pounds and had been trying to do so for more than ten years. She was working as an account executive and between entertaining her clients two or three times a week, going out with her boyfriend on weekends, and occasionally having a glass or two of wine with her dinner, she consumed an average of twenty-four alcoholic drinks a week. The more we talked, the more I realized that Beth viewed having alcohol as essential to her enjoyment of social occasions. I also knew that averaging twenty-four alcoholic beverages each week would make permanent weight loss extremely difficult. I told Beth that although her exercise habits were quite good, she would need to address her weekly consumption of alcohol if she was going to be successful in losing weight. I asked her if she would be willing to cut out alcohol completely for six weeks, at which time we would reintroduce it, but at half of the current amount. I would have liked to see her alcohol consumption reintroduced at an even lower amount than twelve drinks a week, but I felt I was already pushing it with the six-week prohibition period. She surprised me; I fully expected her to start negotiating with me. She didn't. She looked me straight in the eyes and said, "I'll do it."

Beth starting losing weight the second alcohol-free week. After six weeks, she was two pounds away from the weight that she had always wanted to be. She said she didn't want to reintroduce alcohol until she was at her goal weight. Three weeks later, she not only hit her goal weight but went a pound under it. Beth told me that reaching her goal weight was very nice but what was amazing was how her life had changed in many other ways. During those last nine weeks she had received a promotion, she had become closer to her boyfriend than she ever thought was possible, and, most important, she felt that she was so much more in touch with what she wanted in her life.

Beth finally did reintroduce alcohol into her life. She will now have a glass or two of wine whenever she feels like it, but that's it. And she's maintained her goal weight now for two years.

There's no doubt that consuming alcohol makes the weight loss process that much more difficult. So either eliminate alcohol, cut your consumption in half, or reduce it as you feel is best for you. Just remember that the more you restrict your alcohol consumption, the lower your weight will be and the better your overall health will be. You'll also notice that the fitter you become, the more sensitive you'll be to alcohol, making it easier to further cut your consumption.

Simple Ways to Cut Down on Your Consumption of Alcohol

- When you feel like having a drink, try nonalcoholic beverages. Healthy snack foods can also be a substitute. You can also try hot, herbal tea or soup, since having something warm can be a comfort.
- When you feel like having a drink to relax, find alternative activities to do. Take a walk, play a sport, read a novel, take a bubble bath, meditate, or just play soothing music.
- When you do imbibe, use less alcohol in your drinks. You can make a

wine spritzer with sparkling water or cut your hard liquor drinks with water, tonic, or other mixers. Or follow your first drink with club soda with a twist of lime.

- Be sure to have plenty of water and try eating *before* you attend a social event at which you know alcohol will be served. By being full, you'll feel less like drinking once you're there.
- One drink is considered to equal one ounce of hard liquor, one glass (or six ounces) of wine, or twelve ounces (one can) of beer. With that in mind, estimate your average weekly alcoholic drink consumption. If you're not sure of what your normal consumption is, keep an accurate record for one week. You can use the log below to do this. Be sure that the week you choose represents a typical week for you.

WEEKLY ALCOHOL LOG

Date	Number of Alcoholic Beverages
Monday	_____
Tuesday	_____
Wednesday	_____
Thursday	_____
Friday	_____
Saturday	_____
Sunday	_____
Weekly Total	_____
Weekly Target (half of total)	_____

Get with the Program Journal—Phase Two

By now you should have a good idea of what's expected of you in Phase Two. If you're unclear or confused about any of the information discussed this far, please go back and reread it. Use the following checklist to make sure that by now you have:

❑ Read all of the information up through this section at least once and understand it.
❑ Selected at least one, preferably more, aerobic exercise to perform.
❑ Cleared the necessary time in your schedule to exercise.
❑ Taken the time to understand how to exercise in the zone and have practiced doing so.
❑ Determined your weekly alcohol consumption target and have recorded it below (if applicable).

Phase Two Requirements

Water: seven glasses each day
Functional exercises: one set of fifteen, four times per week
Weekly aerobic minutes: a minimum of fifty minutes per week, increasing to seventy-five minutes as you prepare for Phase Three
Limit your consumption of alcohol
Recommended time at Phase Two: one to three months

PHASE TWO—WEEK ONE					
	Water (8-ounce glasses)	Functional Exercises (1 set)	Aerobic Minutes (minimum of 10 minutes)	Number of Alcoholic Drinks	Comments About This Week
Monday					
Tuesday					
Wednesday					
Thursday					
Friday					
Saturday					
Sunday					
Weekly Totals					
Weekly Targets	7	4	50		

PHASE TWO—WEEK TWO

	Water (8-ounce glasses)	Functional Exercises (1 set)	Aerobic Minutes (minimum of 10 minutes)	Number of Alcoholic Drinks	Comments About This Week
Monday					
Tuesday					
Wednesday					
Thursday					
Friday					
Saturday					
Sunday					
Weekly Totals					
Weekly Targets	7	4	50		

PHASE TWO—WEEK THREE

Monday					
Tuesday					
Wednesday					
Thursday					
Friday					
Saturday					
Sunday					
Weekly Totals					
Weekly Targets	7	4	55		

PHASE TWO—WEEK FOUR

Monday					
Tuesday					
Wednesday					
Thursday					
Friday					
Saturday					
Sunday					
Weekly Totals					
Weekly Targets	7	4	55		

PHASE TWO—WEEK FIVE

	Water (8-ounce glasses)	Functional Exercises (1 set)	Aerobic Minutes (minimum of 10 minutes)	Number of Alcoholic Drinks	Comments About This Week
Monday					
Tuesday					
Wednesday					
Thursday					
Friday					
Saturday					
Sunday					
Weekly Totals					
Weekly Targets	7	4	60		

PHASE TWO—WEEK SIX

Monday					
Tuesday					
Wednesday					
Thursday					
Friday					
Saturday					
Sunday					
Weekly Totals					
Weekly Targets	7	4	60		

PHASE TWO—WEEK SEVEN

Monday					
Tuesday					
Wednesday					
Thursday					
Friday					
Saturday					
Sunday					
Weekly Totals					
Weekly Targets	7	4	65		

PHASE TWO—WEEK EIGHT

	Water (8-ounce glasses)	Functional Exercises (1 set)	Aerobic Minutes (minimum of 10 minutes)	Number of Alcoholic Drinks	Comments About This Week
Monday					
Tuesday					
Wednesday					
Thursday					
Friday					
Saturday					
Sunday					
Weekly Totals					
Weekly Targets	7	4	65		

PHASE TWO—WEEK NINE

Monday					
Tuesday					
Wednesday					
Thursday					
Friday					
Saturday					
Sunday					
Weekly Totals					
Weekly Targets	7	4	70		

PHASE TWO—WEEK TEN

Monday					
Tuesday					
Wednesday					
Thursday					
Friday					
Saturday					
Sunday					
Weekly Totals					
Weekly Targets	7	4	70		

PHASE TWO—WEEK ELEVEN

	Water (8-ounce glasses)	Functional Exercises (1 set)	Aerobic Minutes (minimum of 10 minutes)	Number of Alcoholic Drinks	Comments About This Week
Monday					
Tuesday					
Wednesday					
Thursday					
Friday					
Saturday					
Sunday					
Weekly Totals					
Weekly Targets	7	4	75		

PHASE TWO—WEEK TWELVE

	Water (8-ounce glasses)	Functional Exercises (1 set)	Aerobic Minutes (minimum of 10 minutes)	Number of Alcoholic Drinks	Comments About This Week
Monday					
Tuesday					
Wednesday					
Thursday					
Friday					
Saturday					
Sunday					
Weekly Totals					
Weekly Targets	7	4	75		

If you can check off the following statements as being true . . .

❑ I fully understand all of the information contained in Phase Two.
❑ I've fulfilled all of the requirements for Phase Two for at least four consecutive weeks.
❑ I've not begun to lose weight *or* I've lost weight and reached a real plateau.
❑ I've looked at the requirements of Phase Three, and I'm confident I can meet the challenge.

. . . you're ready to move on to Phase Three. Congratulations!

GETTING REAL ABOUT "EMOTIONAL EATING"

If there is a secret to the mystery of permanent weight loss, it is the *complete* elimination of what I call *emotional eating*. If you are like the majority of people who want to lose weight, you almost certainly have struggled long and hard with this issue. Do any of these statements sound familiar?

"Eat this and you will feel better."

"Be a good girl and clean your plate."

"Have a cookie and stop your crying."

"He's a good eater, just like his father."

One of your earliest unconscious lessons was that food equaled comfort. You began receiving your earliest emotional messages as an infant, when you learned that being fed made you feel happy and safe and content, while feeling hungry made your stomach churn and gurgle and caused you to cry.

As you grew up, you may have dealt with various personal stresses as well as traumatic experiences by turning to food for comfort and emotional satisfaction. If so, you are not alone.

Emotional overeating is an epidemic in this country. If you feel you are among this majority, take heart. In Phase Three I'm going to teach you how to regain control over your eating habits and take responsibility— once and for all—for your weight, health, and well-being by coming to grips with the grip of emotional eating.

If you have completed the first two phases of Get with the Program, you are definitely ready to take this step. In the journey to regain your health and well-being, *now* is the time for you to focus your attention on the emotional workout part of the program by flexing your mental muscles in order to get really serious about your personal issues with food.

Eliminating all or most of your emotional eating is the most important thing you can do with respect to how you eat, look, live, and feel. If you consider yourself an emotional overeater, this phase will help you to identify your own personal eating triggers. You will explore and embrace their causes, so that you can gain conscious control over their self-destructive results. It is time for you to finally break free of that vicious cycle of comforting yourself with fattening food and empty calories.

Goals for Phase Three

- Begin to understand the causes of and eliminate your emotional eating.
- Drink a minimum of eight glasses of water each day.
- Increase your functional exercises to two sets of each exercise, five times per week.
- Increase your aerobic exercise to a minimum of 100 minutes per week.
- If you want to progress, increase your aerobic exercise to 125 minutes per week as you prepare for Phase Four.
- Maintain your exercise log.

WHAT IS EMOTIONAL EATING AND HOW CAN IT BE ELIMINATED?

Anytime you eat because of something you are feeling as opposed to physical hunger, it is referred to as emotional eating. This type of eating can occur at any time—at meals, in between meals, at social occasions, or late at night. For many people, emotional eating is the primary reason they have gained weight in the first place. Are you an emotional eater?

Emotional eating is a complex issue, and successfully eliminating this destructive behavior typically requires you to make several changes to one or more aspects of your life. The need for these changes has probably been obvious to you—on one level or another—for quite some time. However, for whatever reason or reasons, you have been unable or unwilling to address these issues. These issues can range anywhere from simply finding creative ways to channel the stress in your life to entering some form of psychological counseling.

Are you an emotional eater? Take the time to answer the following questions.

	Circle Your Answer
Do you eat to comfort yourself in stressful situations?	**Yes No**
Do you eat due to boredom and/or loneliness?	**Yes No**
Do you eat due to problems or turmoil in your life?	**Yes No**
Do you eat due to something (or someone) missing in your life?	**Yes No**

If you answered yes to any of these questions, then emotional eating affects you.

Eliminating all or most of your emotional eating is an essential component to Getting with the Program. It is just as important to your success as, if not even more so than, the challenge of incorporating consistent exercise and a sensible diet plan into your daily routine for life. By eliminating emotional eating, you will not only achieve true weight loss success but will also be giving yourself a life filled with more health and fulfillment than you could ever imagine. But keep in mind that it has taken you a lifetime to weave the threads of overeating into your life, so it will take more than a little time to unravel them as well. Creating positive change in your life can take hard work, painful soul-searching, patience, perseverance, and time.

The rewards of exploring and identifying your inner comfort zones and self-destructive eating issues will benefit and remain with you for the rest of your life.

Emotional eating is invariably tied to one or more other areas of your life: stress at home or at the workplace, boredom or depression, loneliness or disappointment, fear of failure or of success, or deep-seated reasons stemming from emotional trauma that has resulted in an extreme lack of self-love and self-esteem.

I want you to first understand that emotional eating is a coping mechanism—just as a baby soothes herself by sucking on her thumb or a child clings to his raggedy security blanket for emotional self-comfort. Emotional eating also has similarities to workaholism and other forms of addiction, in which negative behaviors help to numb people from the stresses and strains of their lives.

It's a Habit That's Hard to Break

Sometimes life just isn't fair. If emotional overeating is your coping mechanism of choice, you will need to be especially gentle with yourself as you go about the process of eliminating this behavior from your life. For unlike those who suffer from other self-destructive habits, the emotional overeater has an even harder row to hoe because food is an integral part of our lives. You *need* food to live.

You need to acknowledge that being an emotional overeater makes life even harder—just as work does to a chronic workaholic, alcohol does to an alcoholic, or drugs do to a drug addict.

Emotional eating can become an addiction—an addiction to food instead of to drugs, alcohol, cigarettes, sex, or gambling.

How to Begin Eliminating Emotional Eating

- Organize your eating.
- Make eating a conscious activity.
- Learn the difference between physical and emotional hunger.
- Identify the reasons and occasions that you eat out of emotion. Write your thoughts in your journal.
- If you are depressed, consider seeking professional counseling.
- Use the moment of temptation to learn what needs to change in your life.
- Do the hard work of changing your unwanted behavior, one episode at a time.

ORGANIZING YOUR EATING

Let's take a look at the typical American way of eating. Most people skip breakfast, eat a moderate to large lunch on the fly, snack whenever they feel the urge, eat a very large dinner, eat while watching television in the evening, then cap it all off with a late night snack. This is the perfect prescription for gaining weight. Aside from taking all of the conscious pleasure out of eating, most of the calories eaten this way are consumed at the end of the day. Why is this a problem? Calories eaten earlier in the day can raise your metabolism and your energy level to a much greater extent. Foods eaten late in the day are usually more calorie dense, and you're likely to eat more. Instead of being used, these calories are more likely to be stored as fat.

Organizing your meals will help you tremendously in identifying any emotional eating.

> Eat a healthy breakfast.
>
> Eat a moderate lunch.
>
> Have a snack in between lunch and dinner.
>
> Eat a moderate dinner.
>
> Eat a second snack only if you're physically hungry.
>
> Stop eating completely at least two hours before bedtime.

These should be the only times when you eat. Whenever you're tempted to eat outside these meals (and snacks), either it will be due to not managing your meals properly by not eating enough or it's some form of emotional eating. Just by organizing your meals, you're becoming more conscious about what you eat and when you eat it.

By eating this newly conscious way, your consumption of calories will be distributed throughout the day, maximizing your energy level and your metabolism. You will also prevent what is known as an insulin response, which occurs when you eat too many calories at any one sitting. In other words, when you eat one particularly large meal, your body secretes an unusually high amount of insulin. Insulin's job is to take blood glucose out of the bloodstream and deposit it as body fat. And let's face it, when you want to lose weight, this is exactly what you don't want to happen. The ironic part is that many people are under the impression that by skipping breakfast and "saving" those calories for lunch, they are speeding up their weight loss—the opposite is true.

So it all starts with breakfast! If you're not accustomed to eating breakfast, you will need to train yourself to eat this most important meal. When you first start to eat breakfast, you probably won't be hungry for it. This will change as you become accustomed to moving more of the calories that you eat to earlier in the day. Eating breakfast will result in eating less at night and waking up hungrier than you're accustomed to being. This might take a week or a month to occur, but when it happens it's a very good sign.

Once you've gotten into the habit of eating breakfast, your snacks will become an important technique for bridging your hunger in between meals and should help you from overindulging at any one meal. Snacks should be kept anywhere from 75 to 150 calories.

In a perfect world, all three of your main meals would contain approximately the same number of calories. Whether you actually achieve this or not, you must get away from any one meal being excessively larger than the other two.

Again, I can't stress enough how important it is to stop eating at least two hours before bedtime. Late night calories do the most damage because your metabolism is slow. That slight craving for something late in the evening is your body warning you that if you don't feed it, it's going to dip into your fat stores for some energy. Let it! Just go to sleep wanting a little something and let the feeling pass.

One last comment: When your day is done and most of the stresses of life are behind you is when you are the most prone to emotional eating. This is when food can best distract you from feeling something that you were meant to feel. Don't give in; use this critical moment to create a better life for yourself.

Make Eating a Conscious Activity

So much is accomplished by simply organizing all of your eating within three meals and two snacks and shutting down your eating at least two hours before bedtime. By doing this, you are eliminating much of the unconscious eating that can take place throughout the day. Just think of the times that eating is triggered by some external event in your life such as watching television or attending a social gathering. Unconscious eating severely inhibits the weight loss process. In addition, if you organize your eating, each meal becomes an event—something to look forward to! Therefore, you are much more likely to derive pleasure from it, as opposed to guilt.

Eating should be enjoyed. It must also become a conscious act.

When it is, you're naturally more satisfied with it. The "event" of eating and the quality of that event becomes the focus as opposed to the quantity of food consumed. This is why you should think of your meals (and snacks) as events or little celebrations. You should always strive to create a pleasant eating environment by formally sitting down for all of your meals, playing soothing music, burning candles, or inviting interesting people to join you. Successfully planning your meals makes eating something to look forward to and heightens the entire experience.

This is in sharp contrast to how most people eat. Unconscious eating can become a way of life. Eating in front of the television or eating on the run, denies us the pleasure of eating. Be creative and make eating fun.

The Difference Between Physical Hunger and Emotional Eating

Learning to distinguish when physical hunger ends and emotional eating begins is an essential thing you need to do to identify your emotional eating issues and patterns. If you deal with your emotions by using food, you may have actually lost the ability to feel your physical hunger. In order to feel hunger, you must allow yourself to become hungry. That's where Getting with the Program can really help. Just by being more active physically, as you have been doing in Phases One and Two, you will enhance your ability to become physically hungry. Now the challenge will be for you to delay your eating past your normally scheduled mealtime in order for you to experience the actual physical sensation of hunger. Individuals with medical conditions such as diabetes should consult their physician.

When you first begin to do this, it will no doubt cause feelings of anxiety and stress, physical discomfort, or even pain. These are the feelings that typically lead to emotional eating in the first place. These feelings, however, need to be felt and experienced in order for permanent change to occur. If you allow yourself to experience these sensations of discomfort—both physically and emotionally, while identifying their emotional origins—you will gradually begin to fear them less and less. **Dealing with these feelings and allowing them to help you create changes in your life is your path to ultimate freedom.** As you will discover, the moment these uncomfortable sensations first begin to bubble up inside you is the time when you are the closest you can be to identifying what it is that is really "eating" at you emotionally.

In order to relearn how to eat according to the demands of your physical hunger, you need to get into the habit of knowing exactly *why* you're eating *whenever* you eat. In doing so, you will begin to uncover the times that you're eating for reasons other than your physical hunger. Ironically, after they've indulged, most emotional eaters do know that their eating was both excessive and due to something other than hunger.

A technique that I recommend to help you learn the difference between physical hunger and emotional hunger is to keep a journal of the times that you eat excessively or outside of your established meals and snacks. Ask yourself why you're eating. Then simply write about what you're feeling instead of eating. Include anything that you believe contributes to your feelings of hunger and the situation surrounding them. There is space provided for this in your Get with the Program Journal on page 149. Journaling will help you begin to uncover patterns and situations that are associated with your emotional eating and the source of the feelings that contribute to your behavior.

Once you begin to identify your emotional eating triggers and to experience physical hunger on a regular basis, that real hunger will dictate when and how much you eat.

Believe me, eating because of sheer physical hunger is a wonderful experience, especially if you are not used to it. Eating will become an event to be celebrated and savored—not a guilty indulgence. Food will free you to be the best you can be, instead of literally weighing you down. Even so, I remember that when I told this to a good friend she laughed and said half-jokingly, "Hey, if I only ate when I was hungry, I'd sure be missing a lot of meals!"

Exactly my point!

IDENTIFYING THE REASONS AND OCCASIONS THAT YOU EAT DUE TO EMOTIONS

The five most common reasons for emotional eating are:

boredom

stress

loneliness

emotional turmoil or emotional issues (including depression and that caused by early childhood trauma)

filling a void

BOREDOM

Boredom is perhaps the easiest of these to remedy. If boredom is one of the reasons that you frequently use to eat, this is an opportunity to add new dimensions to your life. Anytime that you're tempted to eat out of boredom, contemplate all of the beneficial things you could be doing at that moment. Ask yourself, "What do I want to do?" You might be surprised at the ideas you come up with. Finish a craft project, take piano lessons, learn a foreign language, start your own business. When you are feeling bored and are tempted to raid the refrigerator, one of the best things you can do instead is to exercise. On the verge of devouring the apple pie that you bought to take to the office picnic? That's the perfect time to go out for a long walk, go for a jog, go swimming, or head to the gym. Just get up and move . . . out of your own way.

When it comes to eliminating boredom, you're only limited by your imagination. If you want to make a written list of all the things that you've ever wanted to do or accomplish (besides new ways to exercise!), you can either use the Get with the Program Journal on page 149 or create your own. And the best time to do this is when you're bored.

STRESS

Our lives are more stressful these days than ever before, and food is one of the most common ways that we deal with our stress. Whether it's stress from work, home, children, a significant other, or just the traffic encountered on the way home, stress is part of our lives and it always will be. If stress is a reason that you frequently overindulge, here's some good news: It's one of the easiest reasons to overcome. The first thing you need to do is identify the sources of stress in your life. Write them down in the journal on page 149. Once this is done, you should be able to recognize the sources of stress that can at least be minimized and some that can be eliminated. Just seeing a written list of the things that produce stress in your life tends to minimize their importance and allows you to come up with healthy ways to cope with or eliminate those situations.

If stress is a serious problem in your life, you could refer to one of the countless books on the subject of stress management or enroll in a formal stress-management course at the local university, college, or adult education center in your area.

Exercise is a healthy outlet to deal with that stress when it *does* creep into your life. Make a list of others, such as reading a book, seeing a movie, taking a bubble bath, calling a friend or loved one, scheduling a massage, practicing yoga, or writing a letter—anything that you enjoy doing. Just be sure that whatever you choose acts to reduce, not increase, the amount of stress you are feeling.

Debbie's Story

A few years back, I worked with a commodities broker named Debbie, who needed to be at work by 5:00 A.M. in order to prepare herself for her day on the trading floor. I knew that the key to her weight loss success would be to reduce the amount of stress in her life as well as finding more effective outlets for stress. When I first suggested that she work out for relaxation benefits before her workday started, she chuckled and said, "Right, we could meet at 3:00 A.M.!" I have to admit, I was relieved she wasn't up for that! Instead I started to work on her eating habits.

First we organized all of her eating into a "three meals, two snacks" format. She began eating breakfast for the first time in her life. She also added healthy snacks and worked to eliminate most of the unconscious eating that occurred at her desk. She no longer ate past 8:00 P.M. In addition to these changes, Debbie went into the office a half hour later than usual and meditated at home during this extra time. She also vowed not to bring her work home with her, which significantly cut down on her nervous eating there. Over the course of the next year, Debbie lost thirty-five pounds. There was no doubt that this weight loss was directly related to her eating habit changes, which made her eating more of a conscious activity, as well as her lifestyle changes that removed stress from her life.

LONELINESS

Using food as a replacement for human interaction is an exceptionally easy habit to slip into. What better way to cheer yourself up and to make yourself forget that you are alone on a Saturday night than by plopping yourself in front of the television set with a bottle of soda and a big bag of potato chips, or Chinese food, or pizza, or that irresistible pecan pie . . . with ice cream.

It's no surprise that "comfort food" has become one of our culture's most popular catchphrases. There is nothing quite like a warm bowl of macaroni and cheese or mashed potatoes and gravy to make you forget your isolation. Food has an almost mystical quality of disguising itself as your "friend."

If you find yourself eating out of loneliness, you need to focus on the real reasons behind why you are eating instead of picking up the phone and calling a friend or family member to chat with or making plans to socialize more. When the urge to eat strikes you when you are by yourself and not truly feeling hungry, stop yourself and write down your thoughts in your journal. They may be quite melancholy. That's okay. It's healthy. It's therapeutic. Get real about your feelings. Let them flow and let them go. Don't let food take the place of friends.

Use your newfound personal awareness to expand your social horizons. Keep a list of friends and family members you can call on a moment's notice to help keep your mind off the refrigerator when you're feeling all alone and anxious. Or jump on the Internet and go surfing for Web sites about your favorite hobby or special interests (such as politics, show business, even cooking) in order to connect with like-minded people to chat with. Write a letter to a long-lost friend. Play with your pet (or think about getting one). Make regular appointments to socialize with the favorite people in your life, join clubs, take classes—even join a gym—to increase your odds of making new friends. Remember that loneliness is a choice. It's a situation that you can resolve—not with food, but with personal change and action.

I guess Debbie got used to a less stressful life; since the last I heard from her, she gave up trading commodities, became a personal trainer, and moved to Ohio. But the main point I'm trying to make is that stress can negatively affect your eating habits, but there are unlimited ways to reduce and cope with it once you make the effort.

EMOTIONAL ISSUES OR EMOTIONAL TURMOIL

Emotional issues or turmoil are either temporary situations that crop up in our lives or more chronic conditions of emotional distress. Obviously this category of emotional eating is more complex than the previous three, but the basic intervention remains similar. First, you must identify the emotional issue that is causing the excessive eating. Because the act of eating distances you from feeling emotional distress, resisting the temptation to eat when you're upset will give you a clearer opportunity to identify or clarify what's distressing you. Keeping a journal of emotional eating episodes can be quite helpful in learning not only what the root of your emotional distress is but also what events or situations in your life trigger these episodes. And while some issues can be managed on your own, others require the help of friends, family members, or, in some cases, a professional therapist. Once you identify the cause or causes of emotional distress, a plan for dealing with these emotional issues can be put into motion.

The emotional turmoil of depression is often the result of deep-seated sadness, fear, and anger. **It is one of the most insidious of all the causes for emotional overeating, and it often has its roots in some form of childhood trauma.** It is a condition that should be taken extremely seriously.

In our society, we have been raised to hide our feelings and to put on a happy face. If you find that you are eating to mask your feelings of sadness, fear, or anger, be aware that it is only a temporary salve to your unhappiness. Unfortunately, the habit of emotional eating can begin extremely early in people who have suffered serious blows to their self-esteem, especially when those blows occur in early childhood. Eating is such a strong self-comfort mechanism for many people that it becomes a pattern for the rest of their lives. Many people who deal with this type of emotional eating trigger sometimes trace their emotional eating binges back to a specific traumatic event in their past, be it abandonment, abuse (verbal, physical, and/or sexual), or simply the lack of proper parenting.

If this sounds like you, take heart, and take your time. Find support through your friends, family, or counseling. Explore the origin of your depression. Focus on why you use food to make you feel happy and safe. Examine why you have been resistant to your own health and happiness.

The good news is that support and treatment are available, including therapy and medication. Being conscious of the situation is the first step; don't be afraid to ask for help.

John's Story

During our initial consultation, John told me about his chronic episodes of binge eating. As we began to workout together one day, I asked him why he never sought professional help for his bouts of ravenous eating. He replied, "I just never thought they were that serious and I would always just workout twice as hard the next day to compensate for the episode." We talked about other issues, and John mentioned, almost in passing, that he no longer spoke with his parents. I felt strongly that John needed to discuss his episodes of binge eating with a professional, and he agreed. When he began counseling, John found out that his episodes of binge eating were directly related to his unresolved feelings about his severed relationship with his parents. He started to show better weight loss results almost immediately, but he didn't reach his goal weight until eight months after he renewed his relationship with his parents. The entire process took nearly two years. John had a lot of hard work to do in order to resolve the issues that were related to his binge eating, but the beauty of this process was that John now had a healthier life—emotionally *and* physically.

FILLING A VOID

Companionship, feelings of being appreciated, financial security, feeling safe, feeling a sense of contribution to society, and being able to express and receive love are all things that we seek. When we don't receive these things, we feel something is missing in our lives. Using food to satisfy this emotional hunger is a rather common form of emotional eating, and one of the most difficult causes to overcome.

The first step, which is often the hardest, is to pinpoint exactly what you feel you're missing. Often it's a romantic relationship. But romantic relationships don't always magically appear when you want them to, and a healthy relationship is one in which you don't look to the other person to make you happy.

If eating to fill a void in your life sounds like one of your emotional eating triggers, you must seek out new sources of personal satisfaction and emotional gratification. You must find new activities and relationships that will reinforce your self-esteem and sense of well-being. Participate in volunteer work, sign up for a class to learn how to sharpen your career skills, speak a new language, sail, manage your finances, or grow orchids. Enter bike or running races in your community, based on your level of fitness. Consider the practice of meditation. Yoga is quickly becoming one of the most popular physical and spiritual activities around, and those who practice this ancient form of meditative discipline report a renewed sense of personal harmony and inner peace after each session.

Remember: Eating can be a coping mechanism that allows you to avoid or procrastinate the resolution of emotional issues that negatively affect your life. The issues need to be addressed, not just the eating.

Julie's Story

Julie wanted to lose about fifteen pounds. I had been working with her for about four months and I can say that she was as dedicated with her exercise as anyone I've ever known. She ate a healthy breakfast, a perfect lunch, a small snack in between lunch and dinner, and a perfectly proportioned, healthy dinner. The only problem was that at least two or three times a week, she would eat right before bedtime. And not just a snack. She could devour four or five bagels, a large box of cookies, or just about anything that happened to be available at the time. There was no question where her extra fifteen pounds came from.

As far as I could tell, the binges did not coincide with any other events that were occurring in her life. For whatever reason, she resisted trying any form of counseling. In an attempt to learn more about why she was binging, I asked her when she had first begun this type of eating. About six years ago, she told me. About a week later, Julie was telling me about her first date with some guy. We were laughing hysterically because everything that could go wrong on a first date did go wrong. I was used to these dating stories from Julie, but this one was especially comical. But then I started thinking about it. Julie never went out with the same person more than once, and there was always some funny story about the date. I asked her one day if she was ever in a long-term relationship. She replied, "Oh, yes. I saw Jim for nearly eight years." I asked her when that relationship ended. Julie said, "Oh, six years ago."

It was obvious that Julie's eating episodes were related to her relationship with Jim. Obvious to me, that is. Julie still did not connect her binging to this failed relationship until I asked her *exactly* when the relationship ended and the eating began. She told me that she began her night eating about a month after the breakup. After she said this, she became silent. I could almost see the lightbulb go on above her head.

Seven months after, Julie began to seek professional counseling and she began dating a man on a steady basis. Six months after that they were engaged and making plans to move out East. Julie's eating episodes stopped almost immediately after she felt she had a special person in her life.

Once Julie identified the source of her emotional hunger and what the void in her life was, she was able to look for a way to satisfy it without using food. For Julie, this meant that she had to be open to a new relationship.

If you suspect that you use food to fill a void in your life, take the time to identify what's missing from your life. If you already know what that is, you can begin to immediately direct your energies to bringing more satisfaction into your life or to adopt a new attitude regarding what you're missing. Avoid thinking that what you want can't be obtained. Whatever your needs are, they can be met. You may, however, need to be flexible in the details of your requirements and in how you go about obtaining what you want. The fact that you're making progress toward filling your own needs, and *recognizing* that you're making progress, makes you less susceptible to emotional eating.

USING THE MOMENT OF TEMPTATION AS THE IMPETUS FOR CHANGING YOUR LIFE

Emotional eating usually follows a pattern. Perhaps you're prone to late night eating or overdoing it at social occasions. Start being conscious of when and why you eat. Record your patterns of eating in the journal on page 149 or create your own personal journal. The best time to write is when you're tempted to eat. If this opportunity is missed, then it's still helpful to go back and record the details of the episode. Once your patterns are clear, you'll be better prepared for the critical moment when you become aware of *why* you're emotionally eating in the first place. This critical moment typically occurs *right before* you give in to emotional eating. Be prepared, since this moment frequently carries with it some feelings of discomfort or pain; that's why most people give in to emotional eating in the first place. Those feelings are meant to be felt! Write instead of eating! By eating you're running away.

I want you to look at this moment completely differently than you have in the past. You shouldn't feel guilty or distressed that you feel compelled to eat. It's at this very moment, just before you eat, that your golden opportunity to identify the cause of your emotional eating exists. It can also be an opportunity to change an important aspect of your life. Write down everything that you can about each occurrence, including what you're feeling. Instead of eating, ask yourself the tough question about what's eating you! Write about how you're feeling. Even if you do eat, don't view it as a failure, just one opportunity that was lost. There will be others.

If the Urge Is Overwhelming, Then at Least Eat Wisely

If you do fall prey to the occasional bout of emotional eating, at least try to make sensible snack choices when you head for the kitchen.

Choose	Instead Of
fruit	fudge
yogurt	ice cream
skinless grilled chicken breast	cake
popcorn (unsalted)	potato chips
graham crackers	chocolate chip cookies
freshly cut veggies	candy
soup	pie

You get the picture.

Beginning the Hard Work of Changing Your Behavior

Maybe you've been under the impression that the hard work in the process of improving your health and well-being is in exercising consistently or giving up your favorite unhealthy foods. While these things may be hard at first, they're simply things that need to be done. The real hard work, though, is taking a clear-eyed and objective look at your life and finding the courage to make permanent changes to behaviors that you've probably defended for most of your life. This is what makes permanent change possible—and so powerful!

NEW WORDS TO LIVE BY

- *Stop comforting yourself by stuffing down your feelings of sadness, regret, fear, and frustration with cheeseburgers, pizza, pie, and potato chips.*
- *Stop comforting yourself by numbing yourself from the everyday stresses of work and family life by falling prey to obsessive-compulsive snacking.*
- *Stop comforting yourself by fooling yourself that you can fill a void in your personal or professional life simply with food.*

Think about it this way: At the moment that you're the most tempted to emotionally eat, your true self is crying out for you to change your life!

It is when you have an emotional craving for food that you are the closest to realizing your true feelings. When you choose to eat, you're choosing to mask or deaden your true feelings. In a sense, you are anesthetizing yourself with food and thus missing a valuable opportunity to realize what you really need. With most emotional eaters, this becomes a vicious cycle.

Eliminating emotional eating requires discipline, patience, and a serious commitment to improving your life. And that's the best part about overcoming it: You're invariably forced to take a look at your life in its entirety and make improvements to it that you may not have thought of or have been previously unwilling to make. Acknowledging that you are emotionally driven to overindulge in food is half the battle of gaining control over your weight, health, and well-being. It's not an easy war to win, but the choice to change is all yours, and that choice is a powerful weapon.

When all's said and done, it comes down to what you really want and your ability to impose your will.

Get with the Program Journal—Phase Three

By now you should have a good idea of what's expected of you in Phase Three. If you're unclear or confused about any of the information discussed this far, please go back and reread it. Use the following checklist to make sure that by now you have:

❑ Read all of the information up through this section at least once and understand it.
❑ Start to organize your eating into three meals and two snacks, and stop eating at least two hours before you go to bed.
❑ Create a journal of eating and have a plan to keep it with you.
❑ Prepare yourself for the hard work of looking at and changing your behavior.

Phase Three Requirements

Water: Eight glasses each day
Functional exercises: Two sets of fifteen, five times per week
Weekly aerobic minutes: a minimum of 100 minutes per week
(progressing to 125 minutes as you prepare for Phase Four)
Limit your consumption of alcohol
Limit or eliminate your emotional eating
Recommended time at Phase Three: one to three months

PHASE THREE—WEEK ONE					
	Water (8-ounce glasses)	Functional Exercises (2 sets)	Aerobic Minutes (minimum of 10 minutes)	Number of Alcoholic Drinks	Comments About This Week
Monday					
Tuesday					
Wednesday					
Thursday					
Friday					
Saturday					
Sunday					
Weekly Totals					
Weekly Targets	8	5	100		

PHASE THREE—WEEK TWO

	Water (8-ounce glasses)	Functional Exercises (2 sets)	Aerobic Minutes (minimum of 10 minutes)	Number of Alcoholic Drinks	Comments About This Week
Monday					
Tuesday					
Wednesday					
Thursday					
Friday					
Saturday					
Sunday					
Weekly Totals					
Weekly Targets	8	5	100		

PHASE THREE—WEEK THREE

Monday					
Tuesday					
Wednesday					
Thursday					
Friday					
Saturday					
Sunday					
Weekly Totals					
Weekly Targets	8	5	105		

PHASE THREE—WEEK FOUR

Monday					
Tuesday					
Wednesday					
Thursday					
Friday					
Saturday					
Sunday					
Weekly Totals					
Weekly Targets	8	5	105		

PHASE THREE—WEEK FIVE

	Water (8-ounce glasses)	Functional Exercises (2 sets)	Aerobic Minutes (minimum of 10 minutes)	Number of Alcoholic Drinks	Comments About This Week
Monday					
Tuesday					
Wednesday					
Thursday					
Friday					
Saturday					
Sunday					
Weekly Totals					
Weekly Targets	8	5	110		

PHASE THREE—WEEK SIX

Monday					
Tuesday					
Wednesday					
Thursday					
Friday					
Saturday					
Sunday					
Weekly Totals					
Weekly Targets	8	5	110		

PHASE THREE—WEEK SEVEN

Monday					
Tuesday					
Wednesday					
Thursday					
Friday					
Saturday					
Sunday					
Weekly Totals					
Weekly Targets	8	5	115		

PHASE THREE—WEEK EIGHT

	Water (8-ounce glasses)	Functional Exercises (2 sets)	Aerobic Minutes (minimum of 10 minutes)	Number of Alcoholic Drinks	Comments About This Week
Monday					
Tuesday					
Wednesday					
Thursday					
Friday					
Saturday					
Sunday					
Weekly Totals					
Weekly Targets	8	5	115		

PHASE THREE—WEEK NINE

Monday					
Tuesday					
Wednesday					
Thursday					
Friday					
Saturday					
Sunday					
Weekly Totals					
Weekly Targets	8	5	120		

PHASE THREE—WEEK TEN

Monday					
Tuesday					
Wednesday					
Thursday					
Friday					
Saturday					
Sunday					
Weekly Totals					
Weekly Targets	8	5	120		

PHASE THREE—WEEK ELEVEN

	Water (8-ounce glasses)	Functional Exercises (2 sets)	Aerobic Minutes (minimum of 10 minutes)	Number of Alcoholic Drinks	Comments About This Week
Monday					
Tuesday					
Wednesday					
Thursday					
Friday					
Saturday					
Sunday					
Weekly Totals					
Weekly Targets	8	5	125		

PHASE THREE—WEEK TWELVE

Monday					
Tuesday					
Wednesday					
Thursday					
Friday					
Saturday					
Sunday					
Weekly Totals					
Weekly Targets	8	5	125		

If you can check off the following statements as being true . . .

❑ I fully understand all of the information contained in Phase Three.
❑ I've fulfilled all of the requirements for Phase Three for at least four consecutive weeks.
❑ I feel that I've reached a real plateau.
❑ I've looked at the requirements of Phase Four, and I'm confident I can meet the challenge.

. . . you're ready to move on to Phase Four. Congratulations!

Journal of Eating

_____

_____

_____

_____

_____

_____

_____

_____

_____

_____

_____

_____

_____

_____

_____

_____

_____

_____

_____

_____

_____ **(date completed)** _____

SECURING A LIFE OF HEALTH AND EMOTIONAL WELL-BEING

Congratulations on reaching Phase Four, the final phase of Get with the Program. This phase is all about getting strong, fine-tuning your eating habits, and preparing yourself to be active and healthy for the rest of your life. In this phase, you're going to drink at least nine glasses of water each day. You're going to continue with your stretching exercises, just as you did in Phases One, Two, and Three. But for the rest of the functional exercises, instead of doing two sets of fifteen of each exercise, five times a week, as you did in Phase Three, you'll be doing three sets of fifteen of each exercise, five times a week. You're also going to continue to increase your metabolism by increasing your total weekly aerobic minutes: You will be exercising a minimum of 150 aerobic minutes each week. Then, assuming that you want further results, you will add to your weekly aerobic minutes as you feel you're ready. You're also going to begin the process of strength training. Strength training will maintain or increase your muscle weight, allowing you to burn calories more efficiently. Strength training is a key component in the long-term maintenance of a healthy weight and has the added benefit of combating the effects of age. In Phase Four, you'll also begin to fine-tune your eating habits by increasing your choices of healthy foods while decreasing the unhealthy ones that you consume. Finally, you'll make the adjustments that you feel are necessary in order to continue your healthy way of life. And there you have it!

Goals for Phase Four

- Drink a minimum of nine glasses of water each day.
- Increase your functional exercises to three sets, five times per week.
- Increase your aerobic exercise to a minimum of 150 minutes per week.
- Incorporate strength training exercises into your weekly routine, three times per week.
- Progress your aerobic exercise according to your goals.
- Fine-tune your eating by instituting the "Limit 24-7" nutritional guideline.
- Adjust your program so that you can maintain it for a lifetime.
- Maintain your exercise log.

BECOMING STRONG BY ADDING STRENGTH TRAINING TO YOUR LIFE

Why Should You Train with Weights?

First of all, strength training maintains the muscles that you already have and keeps them active. In many cases it will help you increase your musculature. Since your muscles are your primary calorie burners, maintaining and keeping them active is a highly effective way to reduce and control excess weight. Weight training strengthens your body and allows it to function at a higher level by making you capable of doing more work. I don't just mean allowing you to lift more weight; strength training will increase your ability to perform your aerobic exercise at higher levels as well, which will further decrease your percentage of body fat. You'll also get the aesthetic benefit of toned muscles. But one of the most important yet often overlooked benefits of strength training is in the way it combats two of the most profound effects of the aging process: the loss of muscle and the loss of bone mass (osteoporosis). Strength training is the best way to fight both.

So Why Didn't You Start Strength Training in Phase One?

When you begin training with weights, your appetite increases, sometimes dramatically. I didn't want this to happen too early on in your program, especially if you had negative eating habits. And by not weight training right away, you haven't really lost much in the way of immediate results since all those wonderful benefits of strength training that I just spoke of don't occur overnight. They occur over months and years, not hours and days.

In addition, there are two things that I specifically wanted you to accomplish first. I wanted you to have organized your meals and begun to deal with your issues of emotional eating. Second, I wanted the stabilizing muscles of your body (specifically the muscles of your abdomen, back, shoulders, and lower legs) to be good and strong before you challenge the other muscles and joints of your body. This will greatly improve your performance and your overall results, and it will reduce the likelihood of injury. So now that you're ready, let's get started by learning the basics.

THE BASICS OF STRENGTH TRAINING

There are essentially two different muscular qualities that you'll want to improve through strength training; muscular strength and muscular endurance. And while you could focus on either one of these qualities, both of them will be balanced and enhanced with the Get with the Program strength training progression.

The Essential Eight exercises shown in this section represent a basic strength training program that can be performed at home or in a health club or spa. They are geared to train all of the major muscle groups of your body. They are especially recommended if you wish to lose body fat, improve your overall health, increase your muscular performance, enhance your overall appearance, and work on resisting the effects of age on your body. If you wish to train for and compete in specialized events or develop a particular area of your body, then you'll need a more specialized weight training regimen. If this is the case, you may also want to consult a personal trainer or exercise specialist, who can help you weave such a plan into your Get with the Program routine. I recommend that this person be certified by any one of the following: the American College of Sports Medicine (ACSM), the American Council on Exercise (ACE), or the National Strength and Conditioning Association (NSCA).

Strength training is an entirely different activity than your aerobic workout. Many people make the mistake of trying to make them interchangeable. They're not. They accomplish different goals. Your time spent strength training does not apply toward your weekly aerobic minutes.

However, these two activities can be performed within the same exercise session. Whether you follow your aerobic workout with your strength training routine or vice versa is entirely up to you, but your strength training routine should follow your functional exercises.

There is one similarity between your aerobic workout and your strength training regimen. If you want to show improvement, you must progressively challenge yourself. How effective your strength training regimen is will depend on:

- the number of times a week that you strength train
- the number of repetitions (reps) that you perform
- the amount of resistance (weight) that you use
- the number of sets that you perform
- the types of exercises that you perform
- how aggressively you progress your exercise

How Often Should You Strength Train?

When you strength train, you improve both your muscular strength, which is the ability of your muscles to move a resistance, and your muscular endurance, which is the ability of your muscles to perform exercise (or work) for extended periods of time.

Most studies conclude that when you strength train *once* a week, your muscular strength, for the most part, can be maintained, though your muscular endurance may slightly decline over time. When you strength train *twice* a week, your muscular strength can gradually be improved and your muscular endurance can, more or less, be maintained. But when you train *three* times a week, both your muscular strength and your muscular endurance improve significantly. If you train four times a week, the rate of improvement increases slightly. The Get with the Program progression starts you strength training three times a week in Phase Four, and you simply continue training at this frequency. You'll continue to progress by increasing the amount of weight and the number of sets you perform according to your goals. If you develop a passion for strength training, and you're feeling physically and mentally prepared for it, go ahead and increase your weekly workout days to four.

Repetitions

A repetition is one successful completion of a given exercise. By changing the number of repetitions and the number of sets that you perform, and the amount of weight that you lift, you can influence which of your muscular qualities is stressed. In general, a higher number of repetitions using a relatively lower amount of weight is conducive to building more muscular endurance. To build muscular strength, a lower number of repetitions using a relatively higher weight is used.

To complement your aerobic exercise routine and to enhance both your muscular strength and your muscular endurance, you will do between eight and ten repetitions in a set. If the weight that you select is challenging, this will be effective in significantly increasing both your muscular strength and your muscular endurance.

Amount of Weight Used

Selecting the amount of weight that you use for any strength training exercise should take into account your level of fitness as well as what your goals are. Most personal trainers prescribe a weight that is between 60 percent and 80 percent of your maximum ability, with 70 percent of your maximum ability being the most common prescription. To arrive at this number, a trainer will determine the most weight you can lift at one time, and the prescribed percentage of that weight is calculated. This is an acceptable method, but I personally prefer another. I want you to begin each exercise using a very light weight that you know you can lift. Then increase this weight gradually until you arrive at a weight that makes you fatigued after eight or ten repetitions.

Once you select the amount of weight that you'll use for each exercise and are ready to begin an exercise, be sure to do a warm-up set prior to performing the actual set; this will minimize the risk of injury. The warm-up should consist of four or five repetitions, using about half the amount of weight that you selected.

The Number of Sets That You Should Perform

Sets are groupings of repetitions of the same exercise performed before you take a brief break. You're going to begin Phase Four by performing one set of eight different exercises, three times a week. After about a month, you should consider progressing to two sets of each exercise, three times a week. After another month, you can consider progressing to three sets of each exercise, three times a week. Keep in mind that your progress is completely under your control. If you're not ready to increase the number of sets that you're performing, you don't have to. As always, if you're content with your results, you can stop progressing any aspect of Get with the Program.

If you do decide to perform multiple sets, it's important to limit the amount of your rest in between those sets (your rest interval) to between fifteen and thirty seconds. A common mistake people make is to allow too much time to elapse before starting the next set of exercises. This makes their workout much less effective by allowing the muscle to recover and lessening the training effect.

The Type of Exercises to Use

The Essential Eight exercises described below are to be performed with a set of dumbbells. I find this to be the most effective, cost-efficient way to strength train, plus a set of dumbbells is relatively easy to store. You may prefer to go to a health club or spa and use the equipment they have available. With a minimum of modification, any equipment they may have can be used to perform essentially the eight exercises shown below and achieve similar results. Ask a qualified exercise professional at your facility to customize eight exercises that achieve the same goals as the Essential Eight if necessary.

When performing the Essential Eight, make sure to accurately follow the directions and pictures shown below. This will not only insure that you're getting the results that you want, but will insure your safety as well.

And remember, before you start each exercise, don't forget to warm up.

The Essential Eight Dumbbell Exercises

THE SQUAT

TARGET AREA: UPPER LEGS (quadriceps and hamstrings)

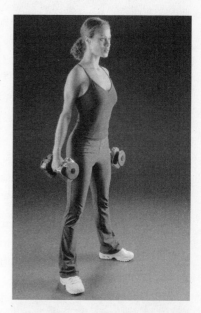

STARTING POSITION

Stand with your feet slightly wider than shoulder-width apart and your toes and knees pointed slightly out. Keep your back straight and your head up. Hold a dumbbell of the appropriate weight in each hand, with your palms facing inward. There should be a slight bend in your knees.

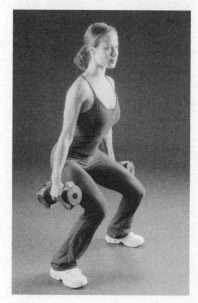

ACTIVE PHASE

Contract your abdominal muscles. Gradually lower your body until your thighs are almost parallel to the floor. *Never* let them go past parallel to the floor. Pause, and then push up from your heels (*not* your toes) before gradually returning to the starting position. Be sure that your torso is leaning only slightly forward throughout the exercise, as shown in the picture below. Control your movement throughout the entire exercise, inhaling on the way down and exhaling on the way up. Continue until the entire set of eight to ten repetitions is complete. If you are performing multiple sets of this exercise, take a deep breath, wait fifteen to thirty seconds, then begin your next set.

THE LUNGE

TARGET AREA: UPPER LEGS (quadriceps, hamstrings, and calves)

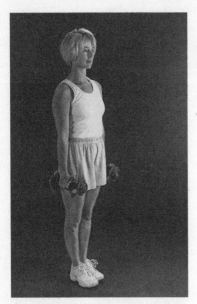

STARTING POSITION

Stand erect with your feet shoulder-width apart. Keep your back straight and your head up. Hold a dumbbell of the appropriate weight in each hand, with your arms down at your sides and palms facing inward. There should be a slight bend in your knees.

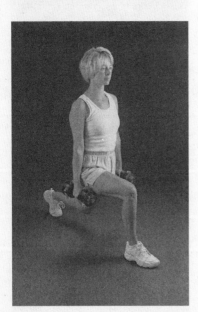

ACTIVE PHASE

Contract your abdominal muscles. Step forward until your front knee is directly above your ankle; never forward of it. Pause, then return to the starting position by pushing off of the front foot. Control your movements throughout the entire exercise, inhaling upon stepping forward and exhaling on the return. Continue until the entire set of eight to ten repetitions is complete. If you are performing multiple sets of this exercise, take a deep breath, wait fifteen to thirty seconds, then begin your next set.

THE CHEST PRESS

TARGET AREA: CHEST AND BACK OF UPPER ARMS (pecs and triceps)

STARTING POSITION

Lie with your back flat on a bench and with your knees bent. Keep your back flat against the bench with little or no arch. Hold a dumbbell of the appropriate weight in each hand, slightly above chest level and with your palms facing forward.

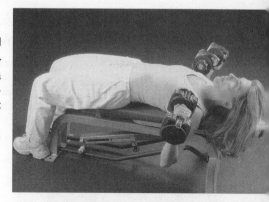

ACTIVE PHASE

Contract your abdominal muscles. Gradually raise both dumbbells up until your arms are fully extended above your chest. Do not hyperextend your elbows. Gradually return the dumbbells back to the starting position. Control your movements throughout the entire exercise, exhaling upon raising the dumbbells and inhaling on the return. Keep your head and back firmly against the bench throughout the entire exercise. Continue until the entire set of eight to ten repetitions is complete. If you are performing multiple sets of this exercise, take a deep breath, wait fifteen to thirty seconds, then begin your next set.

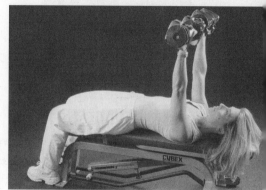

THE SHOULDER PRESS

TARGET AREA: SHOULDERS

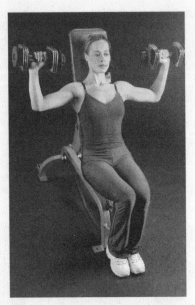

STARTING POSITION

Sit upright on a chair with your back supported and your feet flat on the floor. Keep your back flat against the back of the chair with little or no arch. Hold a dumbbell of the appropriate weight in each hand, slightly above shoulder level and with your palms facing forward. Keep your elbows out to the side.

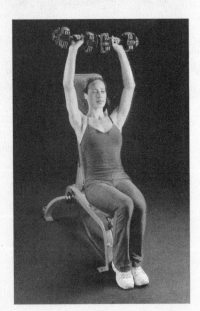

ACTIVE PHASE

Contract your abdominal muscles. Keeping your palms facing forward, raise the dumbbells up and inward until the inside ends of the dumbbells are nearly touching each other and are directly overhead. Do not hyperextend your elbows. Pause, then lower the dumbbells gradually to the starting position. Control your movements throughout the entire exercise, exhaling upon raising the dumbbells and inhaling on the return. Also, be sure to keep your head and back firmly against the back of the chair throughout the entire exercise. Continue until the entire set of eight to ten repetitions is complete. If you are performing multiple sets of this exercise, take a deep breath, wait fifteen to thirty seconds, then begin your next set.

THE BUTTERFLY

TARGET AREA: UPPER BACK (trapezius, latissimus dorsi)

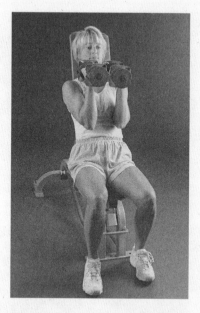

STARTING POSITION

Sit upright on the end of a chair and keep your feet flat on the floor. Keep your back flat with little or no arch. Hold a dumbbell of the appropriate weight in each hand, slightly above shoulder level and with your palms facing inward. Keep your forearms parallel to each other, about four or five inches apart, and your elbows pressed against the front of your body.

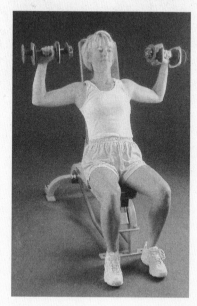

ACTIVE PHASE

Contract your abdominal muscles. Contract the muscles of your upper back while you rotate your forearms back in a semicircle. Keep both dumbbells above shoulder height throughout the exercise. Pause, then gradually return to the starting position. Control your movements throughout the entire exercise, exhaling upon rotating the dumbbells back and inhaling on the return. Be sure to keep your head straight up while looking forward and keep your back straight throughout the entire exercise. It's helpful to visualize squeezing something like a piece of paper with your shoulder blades, and holding it for a split second, then returning to repeat the exercise. Continue until the entire set of eight to ten repetitions is complete. If you are performing multiple sets of this exercise, take a deep breath, wait fifteen to thirty seconds, then begin your next set.

THE DUMBBELL FLY

TARGET AREA: CHEST (pectoralis major, pectoralis minor)

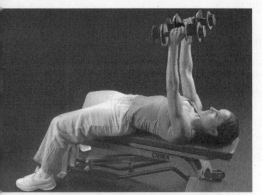

STARTING POSITION

While holding a dumbbell of the appropriate weight in each hand, lie faceup on a bench, with your arms fully extended (not hyperextended) above your chest and your palms facing inward. Keep both feet flat on the floor. Keep your back flat against the bench with little or no arch.

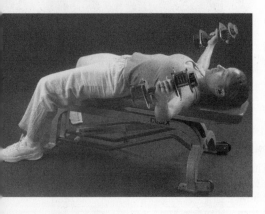

ACTIVE PHASE

Contract your abdominal muscles. Gradually lower the dumbbells, keeping your elbows slightly bent. Continue until your upper arms are parallel with the floor. Maintain a slight bend in your elbows throughout the entire exercise. Pause, then return the dumbbells to the starting position. Control your movements throughout the entire exercise, inhaling upon lowering the dumbbells and exhaling on lifting the dumbbells up to the starting position. Be sure to keep your head and back firmly against the bench throughout the entire exercise. Continue until the set of eight to ten repetitions is complete. If you are performing multiple sets of this exercise, take a deep breath, wait fifteen to thirty seconds, then begin your next set.

THE BICEPS CURL

TARGET AREA: UPPER ARM (biceps)

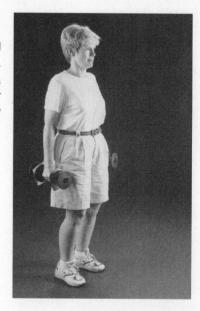

STARTING POSITION

Stand with your feet slightly apart, holding a dumb-bell of the appropriate weight in each hand using an underhand grip. Let your arms hang down at your sides with your palms facing inward. Stand up straight with your knees slightly bent.

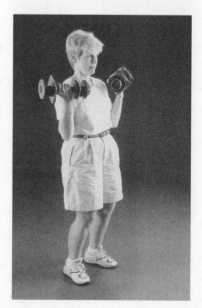

ACTIVE PHASE

Contract your abdominal muscles. Curl the dumb-bells up to your shoulders while twisting your palms so that they are facing you at the top of the exercise. Gradually lower the dumbbells down to the starting position. Maintain your posture throughout the entire exercise and do not allow the dumbbells to "fall" back down. Control your movements throughout the entire exercise, exhaling while lifting the dumbbells up and inhaling on the return to the starting position. Continue until the set of eight to ten repetitions is complete. If you are performing multiple sets of this exercise, take a deep breath, wait fifteen to thirty seconds, then begin your next set.

THE TRICEPS EXTENSION

TARGET AREA: BACK OF UPPER ARMS (triceps)

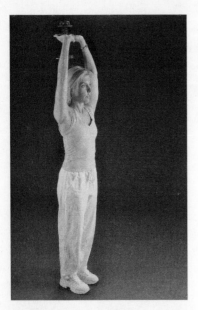

STARTING POSITION

Stand erect with your feet slightly apart and your knees slightly bent. Using an interlocking grip, hold a dumbbell of the appropriate weight above your head with your arms fully extended.

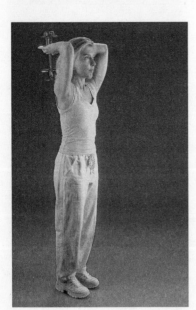

ACTIVE PHASE

Contract your abdominal muscles. Gradually lower the dumbbell back behind your head and neck while keeping your elbows in place above your head. Continue until your forearms are parallel to the floor. Control your movements and maintain your posture throughout the entire exercise. Pause, then gradually raise the dumbbell back up to the starting position. Inhale while lowering the dumbbell down and exhale when raising it up. Continue until the set of eight to ten repetitions is complete. If you are performing multiple sets of this exercise, take a deep breath, wait fifteen to thirty seconds, then begin your next set.

Your Strength Training Progression

How aggressive you are in progressing your strength training program should be based on your ability, your goals, and your level of motivation. Safety should be your primary consideration. There are, however, certain cues that will tell you when you are capable of doing more work. For example, if you're setting your weights properly and working hard, a day or two after you strength train you will notice a slight soreness in the muscles that were exercised. This is not only normal but desired. However, if the soreness is uncomfortable to the point where you don't feel like training on a day you had planned to, the weights that you're using are too heavy and should be lightened. There will come a point when you notice that the same routine using the same resistance no longer produces any muscular soreness and you feel like you could do several more repetitions without a problem. This tells you that it's time to increase the amount of weight that you're using. However, you should increase the weight in the smallest increments possible, typically by two or three pounds. For example, if you're using a three-pound dumbbell for a particular exercise, use a five-pound dumbbell. This is not only to prevent injury, but doing this allows you to see how your body responds to the new weight. Assuming that you want further results and you wish to increase the number of sets that you perform, a general guideline is to work out at least a month using one set, then if you have no muscular soreness, add a second set. Then if after another month or so of doing two sets of each exercise, you want to progress further, and you have no muscular soreness, add a third set.

One final way to increase the intensity of your program is to use a shorter rest interval between your sets, always keeping the interval between the fifteen- to thirty-second guideline. A good rule of thumb is when you first start performing a second set, wait the maximum thirty seconds in between the two sets of each exercise. Keep your rest interval at thirty seconds as long as you're performing two sets. When you first start to train with three sets, continue using a thirty-second interval. After two or three months, you can start decreasing this interval by five seconds at a time. Repeat this pattern until you're at a fifteen-second interval. While it may seem like a small difference to reduce your rest interval by only five seconds, you'll be surprised how much more difficult the next set is when you do so.

There's a strength training log located at the end of this phase to help you keep a detailed record of your program.

Now it's time to fine-tune your eating.

FINE-TUNING YOUR EATING

One of the most common mistakes people make when they attempt to lose weight is radically changing what or how they eat. This usually involves severely limiting the quantity and amount of their food choices. When you do this, you deprive yourself not only of foods that you enjoy but also frequently the nutrients that are essential for your health. And while you may be able to do this for a while, eventually something's got to give! You'll feel deprived physically, or emotionally, or both. And one way or another, this spells the end to your "diet." I strongly believe that the method of eating (and exercise for that matter!) that allows you to lose weight in the first place must, more or less, continue for the rest of your life. That is, you must be successful in maintaining those healthy behaviors for the rest of your life, otherwise any weight lost will eventually return. This is why it's so important to have balance, variety, and moderation in the way you eat.

In order to do this, you will have to think differently about food. No matter who you are, there are choices that you make right now that are good ones and there are choices that need to change. What I want you to do is build healthy eating choices around the way you currently eat while you gradually eliminate unhealthy food choices. It may take a month to make all the necessary adjustments or it may take a year. It should be accomplished on your timetable. That is how change becomes permanent.

Human beings are meant to eat a variety of foods. Severely limiting your food choices is not only boring, it's unhealthy. Your nutritional needs are complex—your body needs a constant and varied supply of calories, carbohydrates, fats, proteins, vitamins, minerals, fiber, water, and electrolytes in amounts and combinations that even a nutritional biochemist would have a hard time keeping up with. Luckily we are naturally attracted to foods that have a variety of colors, textures, and tastes. These preferences become especially keen when your body needs a particular nutrient within a particular food. For example, I don't like carrots—never have. But every so often I find myself craving them. When I crave carrots, my body needs something within this food on a cellular level, such as beta-carotene, vitamin A, or some micronutrient of which I'm completely unaware. On a behavioral level, I'm simply attracted to the bright orange color that is associated with the nutrient or nutrients within this particular food that I need. Nature is truly amazing! In addition to your "nutritional intuition," you have by now a vested interest in your health, well-being, and your weight loss results. Often people who have made exercise a part of their life will quite naturally start choosing healthier foods in more reasonable portions while limiting foods that are not helping their efforts. But simply relying on both your intuition and your good intentions doesn't guarantee you that all of your nutritional needs will be met or that you'll be as consistent as you need to be in order for your weight loss results to continue. In order to help you reach and maintain your goals of health and weight loss, there are four things you need to do each day.

Limit your consumption of fat, especially saturated fat, and "bad" carbohydrates

Eat **2** servings of fruits

Eat **4** servings of vegetables

Eat no more than **7** servings from the whole grain group of foods

Calling these guidelines "Limit 24-7" will help you remember the four things you need to do. Let's first look at limiting fat and "bad" carbohydrates, two culprits that can have negative effects on both your weight loss efforts and your health.

Start by Cutting Out the Fat in Your Diet

Maybe you remember when the first research studies implicated fat—saturated fat in particular—in the incidence of obesity, heart disease, and many forms of cancer. Fat was the enemy and it had to be eliminated from your diet completely. But the truth is that you *need* some fat. Fat aids in your digestion, transports cholesterol, creates hormones, increases your immunity to disease, and helps you realize when you're full. But like most things, too much of it causes problems. It's certainly true that consuming too much fat increases your risk for a variety of diseases and contributes to obesity.

So how much fat should you consume? I don't know exactly, because you have very individual needs. You may require more fat than the average person in order to keep your skin soft or your digestion humming along. Or perhaps you would just feel better with less. You may need to reverse the effects of heart disease, which requires a very low fat diet. Everyone is slightly different and finding out the perfect amount for you takes a little trial and error; most people need somewhere between twenty-five and fifty grams each day. Most, if not all, of this fat should be unsaturated or monounsaturated fats, such as olive oil, canola oil, and safflower oil. Most fat that comes from plants tends to be lower in saturated fat than the fat that comes from animals, like butter and lard. Exceptions to this rule are palm and coconut oil, which are from plant sources but are saturated and, therefore, should be avoided. If you have heart disease, or another medical condition, if you are pregnant or you are a lactating woman, be sure to consult your physician before you make any drastic reductions in your food intake.

So what's the best way to track and limit your consumption of fat?

There are two approaches that I like, and you can pick the one that suits you better. If you like a methodical approach, you could keep a log of your total fat consumption in an average week, then divide this number by seven to get a daily average. Fat grams are now included on virtually all labels. You could also purchase a fat gram counter at your local bookstore or health food store. Your first goal is to be sure that your daily fat consumption is no more than fifty grams a day. Then, by following the recommendations at the end of this section, gradually lower the amount of fat that you consume each day on your own schedule, of course, and give yourself some time to adjust to this new level of fat consumption. Whenever you cut down on anything, your body misses it for a while—*especially* fat. These cravings should eventually go away; when they subside, you can consider making another reduction. However, if after a month or two of this lower fat intake you find that you're rarely satisfied with your meals, you constantly crave foods that are high in fat, or your skin or hair appears dry, you may have cut back a little too much. Just remember to stay within the twenty-five to fifty gram range.

The other approach that I like is more of a commonsense approach to reducing the amount of fat that you consume. Simply begin to gradually cut out foods that are high in fat. The chances are that you already have a good idea how to get most of the saturated fat out of your daily eating, and the following recommendations will give you some new ones. This method is certainly not as structured as the first, but it works quite well for many people. Again, if after the initial adjustment to consuming less fat you find that you're not satisfied with your meals, you constantly crave foods that are high in fat, or your skin or hair appears dry, you may have cut back a little too much.

Pick whichever method is right for you and start getting leaner and healthier today!

Recommendations for Getting Some of the Fat Out

By making just a few adjustments in your behavior, you can drastically reduce the amount of fat that you consume.

- There's a place where you can go that can completely change the way you eat: It's your grocery store. This is where many of your critical decisions are made. Don't fall into the trap of justifying unhealthy choices.

   "I'll only have a little bit of this as a treat."

   "It's really for the rest of my family, I won't have any."

   "Just this once, I'll never buy this again."

   "I'm really buying this for the party next week."

   Don't put unhealthy, high-fat items in your grocery cart! Choose cooking oils such as olive oil or canola oil. Choose lean cuts of meats and poultry. Ignore fatty choices such as bacon, high-fat sausages, brisket, spare ribs, duck, goose, or the fatty cuts of beef. Stay away from highly processed lunch meats such as bologna, salami, corned beef, ham, and pastrami. Choose low- or nonfat milk and low-fat cheeses. Load up on fresh fruits and vegetables.

- Much of the fat that we consume comes from the way that we prepare our meals. Broil, roast, bake, poach, or steam instead of frying. Use oil sprays as opposed to using butter or pouring too much oil in a pan. Many dishes can be prepared without fat or oil. After a little adjustment, you'll notice that more of the natural flavor of the food comes through when you use less fat. You'll be surprised how much fat you can get rid of just by preparing your meals differently.

- When you prepare meat or poultry, trim off all of the visible fat.

- Eat lots of fish! Choose snapper, tuna, mahi-mahi, sole, salmon, monkfish, trout, cod, or bass, and occasionally mackerel, red salmon, and sardines. When you buy canned tuna, be sure it's packed in water, not oil.

- Avoid fried foods. Eventually, you'll even be turned off by too much grease.

- There's a lot of fat hidden in traditional salad dressings. Choose balsamic vinegar or balsamic vinegar mixed with a little olive oil, or buy one of the many low-fat salad dressings that are available. Find low-fat alternatives to gravy and cream sauces, such as low-fat gravy, or tomato- or potato-based sauces. Skim or low-fat milk can be used as a substitute for cream, and low-fat yogurt makes a great substitute for sour cream.

- Desserts can be a source of a considerable amount of fat. Have an arsenal of healthy alternatives for those times that you want a little something sweet after your meal. Fruit, sorbet, ice milk, angel food cake, and fresh berries are all satisfying but low-fat finishes to a meal.

- While snacks are an important way to satisfy your hunger in between meals, they can also add to your total fat count. Toss out potato chips and high-fat treats in favor of pretzels, low-fat soup, or even a baked potato (*without* the butter or sour cream). Air-popped popcorn is good, but hold the butter!

- Restaurants aren't going to be as careful as you are about the way your food is prepared; you can almost always bet your meal is loaded with unnecessary fat. Try to limit the amount of times that you eat out. When you do eat out, pick a restaurant that has some low-fat dishes. Don't be afraid to order off the menu; a good restaurant will want to cater to your needs.

Limiting Sugar and Other "Bad" Carbohydrates

We eat too much sugar. I know I'm guilty. But I got wise and I eat less sugar today than I did a year ago, and much less than I did ten years ago. I've gotten much healthier for it, and so will you. Sugar not only makes you overweight; it contributes to your risk of diabetes, heart disease, and many types of cancer. So let's look for ways to get the sugar and other "bad" carbohydrates out!

The first thing you need to know is that there are carbohydrates that are good for you, and there are those that are not. All carbohydrates are really made up of combinations of simple sugars. The simple sugars are glucose (or blood sugar), fructose, and galactose. When you combine two simple sugars, you get a double sugar (disaccharide). For example, when you combine glucose and galactose, you get the double sugar lactose, which is the sugar found in milk. When you combine glucose with another glucose, you get the double sugar maltose, which is found in beer. When you combine glucose with fructose, you get sucrose. Table honey and brown sugar are both sucrose. Sucrose is one of the "bad" carbohydrates and a primary one that we want *out* of our diet.

When you combine a whole bunch of simple sugars in complex combinations, you get polysaccharides. When a polysaccharide comes from a plant source, it consists of either cellulose or starch. Just think of cellulose as the scientific way to say fiber. As you probably know, fiber is good for you, so you want a lot of this in your diet. The best sources of fiber are in vegetables (especially green leafy vegetables) and fruits. Legumes and whole grain products are also good sources.

Finally, there's starch. Starch is found in some of our favorite foods, such as potatoes, pasta, beans, and rice. Starch has gotten a bad rap through the years. When I was growing up, I can remember people who were on a particular diet saying things like "Can't have any of that, it's got a lot of starch in it!" or "Whoa, that potato is loaded with starch!" And while it's true that too much starch will cause you to gain weight, it's really an important part of a balanced diet.

So besides sucrose, what else is a "bad" carbohydrate? When grains are processed or refined, they're stripped of much of their nutritional value. They become, more or less, empty calories, which we want to avoid. White bread, white rice, white flour, and many pastas are in this category. What you want are whole grain breads, whole grain cereals, brown or whole grain rice, and whole grain pastas. These products may be harder to find and more expensive, but your health is well worth it.

To limit your consumption of "bad" carbohydrates, the commonsense approach is the way to go. Take some time to familiarize yourself with the following list. Start to eliminate those foods you can do without and replace them with healthier choices. Before you know it, the "bad" carbs will be gone from your life. If you need some motivation, check off the "bad" carbs that you currently consume, then pick a target date to remove each from your life. You could pick one "bad" carb per month that you're going to completely eliminate. Personally, I prefer a gradual reduction in "bad" carbohydrates. This will help you to avoid the feelings of being deprived (a common side effect of cutting out your favorite sugary treats all at once). When this process is complete (this could take a year—and that's fine!), you'll be left with only those "bad" carbohydrates that you feel would be difficult (if not impossible!) to live without. At that point, you could even decide that some of those could be slightly reduced.

"Bad" Carbohydrates	Elimination or Reduction Date
❏ table (refined) sugar	_____
❏ sugary cereals	_____
❏ soda	_____
❏ candy	_____

❑ cake   _____

❑ pie   _____

❑ white flour   _____

Processed grain products, such as:

❑ pastas (made with white or refined flour)_____

❑ white rice   _____

❑ white bread   _____

Healthy Choices	**"To Add" Target Date**
❑ whole grain, sugar-free cereals	_____
❑ beans/legumes	_____
❑ whole grain breads	_____
❑ whole grain pastas	_____
❑ whole grain rice	_____
❑ brown rice	_____
❑ fruits	_____
❑ vegetables	_____

RECOMMENDATIONS FOR LIMITING "BAD" CARBOHYDRATES

- Choose whole grain pasta, whole grain bread, and whole grain rice instead of their processed counterparts.
- Take the time to know what you're eating; get in the habit of reading labels. Some products you thought contained a little sugar may be loaded with it. Cereals are a good example; there are only a handful that don't have added refined sugar.
- Cookies, cakes, and frozen desserts (even these labeled "low fat") are usually packed with sugar. If you're not willing to eliminate dessert, at least choose fruit, or sorbet made without sugar.
- Break the soda habit. Soda is almost pure sugar! Water and fresh fruit juices are much better choices. Be sure that any fruit juices you drink are 100 percent pure fruit juice!

Eat 2 Servings of Fruit Each Day

I know, while growing up you always heard that you should eat an apple a day, but here I am asking you to eat two. Well, I guess that's inflation for you. Eating two servings of fruit each day is one of the healthiest things you can do, and it's also one of the easiest. Fruits come in all shapes and sizes, tastes and textures. You'll never get bored, so get on board!

We eat, first and foremost, to satisfy our nutritional needs. If your basic needs are met with nutrient-rich foods, you not only need to eat less to satisfy your nutritional needs, but you'll begin to crave less food. Fruits are nutrient-rich foods; they contain water, vitamins, fiber, and minerals. I do, however, want you to keep in mind that fruits contain the sugar fructose and can contain a fair amount of calories. Two servings of fruit a day is perfect, three is fine. Eating more than three servings of fruit a day is not necessary and only winds up contributing to excess calories. Your two fruits a day will nicely complement the nutritional value that you get from eating your vegetables.

The list below can give you some new ideas that will expand your fruit horizons. Check off the fruits you've tried; then try new ones and check those off. I'm still trying to complete my list. I just need a prickly pear and a gooseberry, and I'll be done!

Note that fruit juice also counts as a fruit, as long as it is 100 percent pure fruit juice—not the type that contains sugar or corn syrup. Dried, canned, and processed fruits are not your best choices and are therefore not listed.

- ❑ apples
  - ❑ Granny Smith
  - ❑ McIntosh
  - ❑ Red Delicious
- ❑ apple juice
- ❑ applesauce
- ❑ apricot juice (only 100 percent pure)
- ❑ apricots
- ❑ avocado
  - ❑ California
  - ❑ Florida
- ❑ bananas
- ❑ blackberries
- ❑ blueberries

- ❑ boysenberries
- ❑ breadfruit
- ❑ cantaloupe
- ❑ casaba melon
- ❑ cherries
  - ❑ sour
  - ❑ sweet
- ❑ coconut
- ❑ crab apples
- ❑ cranberries
- ❑ cranberry juice (only 100 percent pure)
- ❑ cranberry sauce
- ❑ currants
- ❑ dates
- ❑ gooseberries
- ❑ grapefruit
- ❑ grapefruit juice (only 100 percent pure)
- ❑ grape juice (only 100 percent pure)
- ❑ grapes
  - ❑ Concord
  - ❑ Emperor
  - ❑ Thompson
- ❑ guava juice (only 100 percent pure)
- ❑ guavas
- ❑ honeydew melon
- ❑ kiwifruit
- ❑ kumquats
- ❑ lemons
- ❑ limes
- ❑ lime juice (only 100 percent pure)
- ❑ loganberries
- ❑ mangoes
- ❑ mango juice (only 100 percent pure)
- ❑ mulberries
- ❑ nectarines
- ❑ orange juice (only 100 percent pure)
- ❑ oranges
- ❑ papaya juice (only 100 percent pure)
- ❑ papayas

- ❑ passion fruit
- ❑ passion fruit juice (only 100 percent pure)
- ❑ peach juice (only 100 percent pure)
- ❑ peaches
- ❑ pear juice (only 100 percent pure)
- ❑ pears
- ❑ persimmons
- ❑ pineapple juice (only 100 percent pure)
- ❑ pineapples
- ❑ plantains
- ❑ plums
- ❑ pomegranate pulp
- ❑ prickly pears
- ❑ prune juice (only 100 percent pure)
- ❑ prunes
- ❑ quinces
- ❑ raisins
- ❑ raspberries
  - ❑ black
  - ❑ red
- ❑ rhubarb
- ❑ strawberries
- ❑ tangerines
- ❑ watermelon

One serving of fruit equals:
1 medium-size apple, orange, pear, peach, grapefruit,
  or apricot
1 cup of grapes
1 six-ounce glass of fruit juice
1 cup of strawberries, raspberries, blackberries, or boysenberries
1 banana

Eat 4 Servings of Vegetables Each Day

When it comes to nutrition, nothing beats vegetables. They're loaded with vitamins, minerals, water, and fiber, and they fill you up. Their contribution to both your health and weight loss efforts can't be questioned. Just be sure to get in your four a day, even five if you want, and let 'em go to work for you. Even though you can count frozen vegetables toward your vegetable quota, fresh veggies are a far better choice and worth the little bit of extra effort. Canned vegetables have a much lower nutritional value than either frozen or fresh, and I'd avoid them completely. Check off the vegetables that you've tried; experiment with those that you've never had.

- ❏ alfalfa sprouts
- ❏ artichoke hearts
- ❏ artichokes
- ❏ asparagus
- ❏ bamboo shoots
- ❏ beans
    - ❏ green
    - ❏ snap
    - ❏ yellow
- ❏ beet greens
- ❏ beets
- ❏ bok choy
- ❏ broccoflower
- ❏ broccoli
- ❏ broccoli rabe
- ❏ brussels sprouts
- ❏ cabbage
    - ❏ Chinese
    - ❏ red
    - ❏ white
- ❏ carrots
- ❏ cauliflower
- ❏ celery
- ❏ collard greens
- ❏ corn (white)
- ❏ corn (yellow)
- ❏ cucumbers
- ❏ eggplant
- ❏ endive (Belgian)
- ❏ escarole
- ❏ fennel
- ❏ garlic

- ❑ gingerroot
- ❑ greens
  - ❑ beet
  - ❑ collard
  - ❑ dandelion
  - ❑ mustard
  - ❑ turnip
- ❑ Jerusalem artichoke
- ❑ kale
- ❑ kelp (seaweed)
- ❑ kohlrabi
- ❑ leeks
- ❑ lettuce
  - ❑ butterhead
  - ❑ crisphead
  - ❑ loose leaf
  - ❑ mesclun
- ❑ mushrooms
  - ❑ portabella
  - ❑ shiitake
  - ❑ wild
- ❑ okra
- ❑ onions
- ❑ parsnips
- ❑ peas
  - ❑ black-eyed
  - ❑ green
  - ❑ snow
  - ❑ sugar snap
- ❑ potatoes
- ❑ pumpkins
- ❑ radishes
- ❑ rutabagas
- ❑ sauerkraut
- ❑ scallions
- ❑ shallots
- ❑ squash
  - ❑ acorn
  - ❑ butternut

❑ Hubbard
❑ spaghetti
❑ summer (several types)
❑ zucchini
❑ spinach
❑ succotash
❑ Swiss chard
❑ taro
❑ tomatoes (all types)
❑ turnips
❑ water chestnuts
❑ watercress
❑ zucchini

One serving of vegetables equals:

The amount of lettuce, tomato, and onion you would put on a sandwich

½ cup of raw or cooked squash, corn, broccoli, green beans, or cauliflower

1 cup of salad greens

6 ounces or ¾ cup of tomato or carrot juice

Eat a Maximum of 7 Servings from the Grain Group Each Day

You could, if you want to, refer to this group as the *whole* grain group since your best food choices are whole grains, including whole grain breads, cereals, rice, and pastas. Technically, any product containing flour, such as cookies, cakes, pastries, and pies, *could* be considered a part of this group. But you know that these products need to be limited (or eliminated) from your diet, and since they don't positively contribute to your nutritional needs, making them one of your seven daily choices robs you of nutrition. When you do allow yourself one of these indulgences, don't count them in your grain quota. Simply consider it an occasional treat. Just don't treat yourself too frequently!

Pretzels are considered to be in the grain group. They make a great snack, especially the ones that contain no fat and that are made with whole wheat flour.

Just a Few "Grain" Recommendations

- Try to limit your bread servings to three or less a day. If you have a sandwich, it counts as two servings of bread.
- Gradually start replacing processed grains with whole grains, one product at a time. Choose oatmeal over cream of wheat; whole wheat pasta over pasta made with white flour; kasha, barley, or brown rice over white rice. You can even find whole wheat couscous.
- When you go out to eat, don't allow the bread basket to sit on the table. If you want bread, simply ask the person waiting on you to bring a slice or one roll with your meal.

One serving of grain equals:
1 slice of bread
½ cup of cooked cereal, rice, or pasta
1 ounce of breakfast cereal
1 ounce of pretzels (about one large pretzel)

Keeping a Record of Your Eating

It's a good idea to keep a record of your eating when you first begin to follow the "Limit 24-7" eating guideline (there is space in your Get with the Program journal on page 182). Remember that you do not have to be perfect in your eating, just consistent. Consistently good, that is! When you fill in your journal, simply place a check mark on the days of the week that you meet all four guidelines. Again, they are:

> **Limit** your consumption of fat, especially saturated fat and "bad" carbohydrates
>
> Eat **2** servings of fruits
>
> Eat **4** servings of vegetables
>
> Eat no more than **7** servings from the whole grain group of foods

Your weekly goal in Phase Four is to meet all four of the "Limit 24-7" guidelines, a minimum of five times per week.

A Perfect Eating Day

Breakfast
1 healthy stack of potato pancakes
8-ounce glass of grapefruit or orange juice
Cup of herbal tea

Lunch
Bowl of turkey and red bean soup
1 veggie burger
8-ounce glass of skim or 1% milk

Snack
1 ounce of pretzels with mustard

Dinner
Pan-seared fillet of tilapia with mango salsa and lentil pancake
1 cup of snap beans
1 cup of brown or wild rice
1 slice of French bread, lightly brushed with olive oil
8-ounce glass of water with lemon wedge

Snack
1 cup of mixed berries (strawberries, raspberries, boysenberries)

Total servings

Fruit group	2
Vegetable group	4
Grain group (bread, cereal, rice, pasta)	6

INVESTING IN YOURSELF FOR THE REST OF YOUR LIFE

Always remember that your best investment is in yourself. There's no better feeling than working hard toward a goal and seeing it materialize. You have every right to feel good about your accomplishments on the journey of health and fitness that you've taken. Think to your future. If there's an aspect of the program that you honestly feel you can't perform each week going forward, now is the time to adjust it to fit your needs, goals, and life. Remember that all of these good things you do for yourself each day need to be maintained, if not improved upon, for the rest of your life. And while you've been challenged right up until now, the *real* challenge is to make all of these positive changes permanent. You've made it this far and I know, going forward, you're up to the task.

I'd like to leave you with some advice. It comes from years of observing many people take this journey to improve the quality of their lives. Caring for yourself is a daily process. Each day of your life, you wake up and make the choice to either elevate yourself, stay just as you are, or slide backwards—in every area of your life. There's no question that you're going to have good days and not so good days, but what's important are the choices you *consistently* make. This dictates whether your momentum is in reverse or moving positively in the direction of your goals. We need to remember that we create ourselves by the choices we make. And while each of us is blessed with our individual strengths and weaknesses, what we create with that which we have is what is ultimately meaningful.

Get with the Program Journal—Phase Four

By now you should have a good idea of what's expected of you in Phase Four. If you're unclear or confused about any of the information discussed this far, please go back and reread it. Use the following checklist to make sure that by now you have:

❑ Read all of the information up through this section at least once and understand it.
❑ Practiced each of the Essential Eight strength training exercises.
❑ Selected the appropriate amount of weight to be used for each of the Essential Eight exercises.
❑ Learned the "Limit 24-7" guideline and are prepared to institute it.
❑ Taken the time to look at your eating choices and know what needs to change.
❑ Made any adjustments to your program and your life so that you are confident that you can maintain your healthy way of life—for good.

Phase Four Requirements

Water: nine glasses each day
Functional exercises: three sets of fifteen, five times per week
Weekly aerobic minutes: a minimum of 150 minutes per week (progress your aerobic minutes according to your goals)
Strength training: Essential Eight exercises, three times per week (one set to start, progressing to three sets based on your goals)
Limit your consumption of alcohol
Limit or eliminate your emotional eating
Institute the "Limit 24-7" guideline of eating: minimum of five times per week
Recommended time at Phase Four: the rest of your life!

PHASE FOUR—WEEK ONE

	Water (8-ounce glasses)	Functional Exercises (3 sets)	Aerobic Minutes (minimum of 10 minutes)	Number of Alcoholic Drinks	Strength Training (sessions)	"Limit 24-7" (all four)	Comments About This Week
Monday							
Tuesday							
Wednesday							
Thursday							
Friday							
Saturday							
Sunday							
Weekly Totals							
Weekly Targets	9	5	150		3	5	

PHASE FOUR—WEEK TWO

Monday							
Tuesday							
Wednesday							
Thursday							
Friday							
Saturday							
Sunday							
Weekly Totals							
Weekly Targets	9	5	150		3	5	

PHASE FOUR—WEEK THREE

Monday							
Tuesday							
Wednesday							
Thursday							
Friday							
Saturday							
Sunday							
Weekly Totals							
Weekly Targets	9	5	155		3	5	

PHASE FOUR—WEEK FOUR

	Water (8-ounce glasses)	Functional Exercises (3 sets)	Aerobic Minutes (minimum of 10 minutes)	Number of Alcoholic Drinks	Strength Training (sessions)	"Limit 24-7" (all four)	Comments About This Week
Monday							
Tuesday							
Wednesday							
Thursday							
Friday							
Saturday							
Sunday							
Weekly Totals							
Weekly Targets	9	5	155		3	5	

PHASE FOUR—WEEK FIVE

Monday							
Tuesday							
Wednesday							
Thursday							
Friday							
Saturday							
Sunday							
Weekly Totals							
Weekly Targets	9	5	160		3	5	

PHASE FOUR—WEEK SIX

Monday							
Tuesday							
Wednesday							
Thursday							
Friday							
Saturday							
Sunday							
Weekly Totals							
Weekly Targets	9	5	165		3	5	

PHASE FOUR—WEEK SEVEN

	Water (8-ounce glasses)	Functional Exercises (3 sets)	Aerobic Minutes (minimum of 10 minutes)	Number of Alcoholic Drinks	Strength Training (sessions)	"Limit 24-7" (all four)	Comments About This Week
Monday							
Tuesday							
Wednesday							
Thursday							
Friday							
Saturday							
Sunday							
Weekly Totals							
Weekly Targets	9	5	165		3	5	

PHASE FOUR—WEEK EIGHT

Monday							
Tuesday							
Wednesday							
Thursday							
Friday							
Saturday							
Sunday							
Weekly Totals							
Weekly Targets	9	5	165		3	5	

PHASE FOUR—WEEK NINE

Monday							
Tuesday							
Wednesday							
Thursday							
Friday							
Saturday							
Sunday							
Weekly Totals							
Weekly Targets	9	5	170		3	5	

PHASE FOUR—WEEK TEN

	Water (8-ounce glasses)	Functional Exercises (3 sets)	Aerobic Minutes (minimum of 10 minutes)	Number of Alcoholic Drinks	Strength Training (sessions)	"Limit 24-7" (all four)	Comments About This Week
Monday							
Tuesday							
Wednesday							
Thursday							
Friday							
Saturday							
Sunday							
Weekly Totals							
Weekly Targets	9	5	170		3	5	

PHASE FOUR—WEEK ELEVEN

Monday							
Tuesday							
Wednesday							
Thursday							
Friday							
Saturday							
Sunday							
Weekly Totals							
Weekly Targets	9	5	175		3	5	

PHASE FOUR—WEEK TWELVE

Monday							
Tuesday							
Wednesday							
Thursday							
Friday							
Saturday							
Sunday							
Weekly Totals							
Weekly Targets	9	5	175		3	5	

PHASE FOUR—MAINTENANCE

	Water (8-ounce glasses)	Functional Exercises (3 sets)	Aerobic Minutes (minimum of 10 minutes)	Number of Alcoholic Drinks	Strength Training (sessions)	"Limit 24-7" (all four)	Comments About This Week
Monday							
Tuesday							
Wednesday							
Thursday							
Friday							
Saturday							
Sunday							
Weekly Totals							
Weekly Targets*							

* Your maintenance targets are to be adjusted according to your goals.

Strength Training Log

Starting Date _____

Exercise	Target Area	Set	Week # 1 Day 1 1	2	3	Day 2 1	2	3	Day 3 1	2	3	Week # 2 Day 1 1	2	3	Day 2 1	2	3	Day 3 1	2	3
Squat	Quads/Hams/Gluts	Wt																		
		Reps																		
Lunge	Quads/Hams/Calves	Wt																		
		Reps																		
Chest Press	Chest/Triceps	Wt																		
		Reps																		
Shoulder Press	Shoulders	Wt																		
		Reps																		
Butterfly	Lats/Traps	Wt																		
		Reps																		
Dumbbell Fly	Chest	Wt																		
		Reps																		
Biceps Curl	Biceps	Wt																		
		Reps																		
Triceps Ext.	Triceps	Wt																		
		Reps																		
		Wt																		
		Reps																		
		Wt																		
		Reps																		
		Wt																		
		Reps																		
		Wt																		
		Reps																		
		Wt																		
		Reps																		
		Wt																		
		Reps																		

Comments about these two weeks

_____

_____

_____

_____

Strength Training Log

Exercise	Target Area	Set	Week # 3 Day 1 1 2 3	Day 2 1 2 3	Day 3 1 2 3	Week # 4 Day 1 1 2 3	Day 2 1 2 3	Day 3 1 2 3
Squat	Quads/Hams/Gluts	Wt						
		Reps						
Lunge	Quads/Hams/Calves	Wt						
		Reps						
Chest Press	Chest/Triceps	Wt						
		Reps						
Shoulder Press	Shoulders	Wt						
		Reps						
Butterfly	Lats/Traps	Wt						
		Reps						
Dumbbell Fly	Chest	Wt						
		Reps						
Biceps Curl	Biceps	Wt						
		Reps						
Triceps Ext.	Triceps	Wt						
		Reps						
		Wt						
		Reps						
		Wt						
		Reps						
		Wt						
		Reps						
		Wt						
		Reps						
		Wt						
		Reps						
		Wt						
		Reps						

Comments about these two weeks

Strength Training Log

Exercise	Target Area	Set	Week # 5 Day 1			Day 2			Day 3			Week # 6 Day 1			Day 2			Day 3		
			1	2	3	1	2	3	1	2	3	1	2	3	1	2	3	1	2	3
Squat	Quads/Hams/Gluts	Wt																		
		Reps																		
Lunge	Quads/Hams/Calves	Wt																		
		Reps																		
Chest Press	Chest/Triceps	Wt																		
		Reps																		
Shoulder Press	Shoulders	Wt																		
		Reps																		
Butterfly	Lats/Traps	Wt																		
		Reps																		
Dumbbell Fly	Chest	Wt																		
		Reps																		
Biceps Curl	Biceps	Wt																		
		Reps																		
Triceps Ext.	Triceps	Wt																		
		Reps																		
		Wt																		
		Reps																		
		Wt																		
		Reps																		
		Wt																		
		Reps																		
		Wt																		
		Reps																		
		Wt																		
		Reps																		
		Wt																		
		Reps																		

Comments about these two weeks

Strength Training Log

Exercise	Target Area	Set	Week # 7 Day 1 1 2 3	Day 2 1 2 3	Day 3 1 2 3	Week # 8 Day 1 1 2 3	Day 2 1 2 3	Day 3 1 2 3
Squat	Quads/Hams/Gluts	Wt						
		Reps						
Lunge	Quads/Hams/Calves	Wt						
		Reps						
Chest Press	Chest/Triceps	Wt						
		Reps						
Shoulder Press	Shoulders	Wt						
		Reps						
Butterfly	Lats/Traps	Wt						
		Reps						
Dumbbell Fly	Chest	Wt						
		Reps						
Biceps Curl	Biceps	Wt						
		Reps						
Triceps Ext.	Triceps	Wt						
		Reps						
		Wt						
		Reps						
		Wt						
		Reps						
		Wt						
		Reps						
		Wt						
		Reps						
		Wt						
		Reps						
		Wt						
		Reps						

Comments about these two weeks

_____

_____

_____

_____

Strength Training Log

Exercise	Target Area	Set	Week # 9 Day 1 1 2 3	Week # 9 Day 2 1 2 3	Week # 9 Day 3 1 2 3	Week # 10 Day 1 1 2 3	Week # 10 Day 2 1 2 3	Week # 10 Day 3 1 2 3
Squat	Quads/Hams/Gluts	Wt						
		Reps						
Lunge	Quads/Hams/Calves	Wt						
		Reps						
Chest Press	Chest/Triceps	Wt						
		Reps						
Shoulder Press	Shoulders	Wt						
		Reps						
Butterfly	Lats/Traps	Wt						
		Reps						
Dumbbell Fly	Chest	Wt						
		Reps						
Biceps Curl	Biceps	Wt						
		Reps						
Triceps Ext.	Triceps	Wt						
		Reps						
		Wt						
		Reps						
		Wt						
		Reps						
		Wt						
		Reps						
		Wt						
		Reps						
		Wt						
		Reps						
		Wt						
		Reps						

Comments about these two weeks

_____

_____

_____

_____

Strength Training Log

Exercise	Target Area	Set	Week # 11									Week # 12								
			Day 1			Day 2			Day 3			Day 1			Day 2			Day 3		
			1	2	3	1	2	3	1	2	3	1	2	3	1	2	3	1	2	3
Squat	Quads/Hams/Gluts	Wt																		
		Reps																		
Lunge	Quads/Hams/Calves	Wt																		
		Reps																		
Chest Press	Chest/Triceps	Wt																		
		Reps																		
Shoulder Press	Shoulders	Wt																		
		Reps																		
Butterfly	Lats/Traps	Wt																		
		Reps																		
Dumbbell Fly	Chest	Wt																		
		Reps																		
Biceps Curl	Biceps	Wt																		
		Reps																		
Triceps Ext.	Triceps	Wt																		
		Reps																		
		Wt																		
		Reps																		
		Wt																		
		Reps																		
		Wt																		
		Reps																		
		Wt																		
		Reps																		
		Wt																		
		Reps																		
		Wt																		
		Reps																		

Comments about these two weeks

_____

_____

_____

_____

Strength Training Log

Exercise	Target Area	Set	Week # 13 Day 1			Day 2			Day 3			Week # 14 Day 1			Day 2			Day 3		
			1	2	3	1	2	3	1	2	3	1	2	3	1	2	3	1	2	3
Squat	Quads/Hams/Gluts	Wt																		
		Reps																		
Lunge	Quads/Hams/Calves	Wt																		
		Reps																		
Chest Press	Chest/Triceps	Wt																		
		Reps																		
Shoulder Press	Shoulders	Wt																		
		Reps																		
Butterfly	Lats/Traps	Wt																		
		Reps																		
Dumbbell Fly	Chest	Wt																		
		Reps																		
Biceps Curl	Biceps	Wt																		
		Reps																		
Triceps Ext.	Triceps	Wt																		
		Reps																		
		Wt																		
		Reps																		
		Wt																		
		Reps																		
		Wt																		
		Reps																		
		Wt																		
		Reps																		
		Wt																		
		Reps																		
		Wt																		
		Reps																		

Comments about these two weeks

_____

_____

_____

_____

Strength Training Log

Exercise	Target Area	Set	Week # 15 Day 1 1 2 3	Day 2 1 2 3	Day 3 1 2 3	Week # 16 Day 1 1 2 3	Day 2 1 2 3	Day 3 1 2 3
Squat	Quads/Hams/Gluts	Wt						
		Reps						
Lunge	Quads/Hams/Calves	Wt						
		Reps						
Chest Press	Chest/Triceps	Wt						
		Reps						
Shoulder Press	Shoulders	Wt						
		Reps						
Butterfly	Lats/Traps	Wt						
		Reps						
Dumbbell Fly	Chest	Wt						
		Reps						
Biceps Curl	Biceps	Wt						
		Reps						
Triceps Ext.	Triceps	Wt						
		Reps						
		Wt						
		Reps						
		Wt						
		Reps						
		Wt						
		Reps						
		Wt						
		Reps						
		Wt						
		Reps						
		Wt						
		Reps						

Comments about these two weeks

_____

_____

_____

_____

Strength Training Log

Exercise	Target Area	Set	Week # 17 Day 1 1 2 3	Day 2 1 2 3	Day 3 1 2 3	Week # 18 Day 1 1 2 3	Day 2 1 2 3	Day 3 1 2 3
Squat	Quads/Hams/Gluts	Wt						
		Reps						
Lunge	Quads/Hams/Calves	Wt						
		Reps						
Chest Press	Chest/Triceps	Wt						
		Reps						
Shoulder Press	Shoulders	Wt						
		Reps						
Butterfly	Lats/Traps	Wt						
		Reps						
Dumbbell Fly	Chest	Wt						
		Reps						
Biceps Curl	Biceps	Wt						
		Reps						
Triceps Ext.	Triceps	Wt						
		Reps						
		Wt						
		Reps						
		Wt						
		Reps						
		Wt						
		Reps						
		Wt						
		Reps						
		Wt						
		Reps						
		Wt						
		Reps						

Comments about these two weeks

_____

_____

_____

_____

Strength Training Log

Exercise	Target Area	Set	Week # 19									Week # 20								
			Day 1			Day 2			Day 3			Day 1			Day 2			Day 3		
			1	2	3	1	2	3	1	2	3	1	2	3	1	2	3	1	2	3
Squat	Quads/Hams/Gluts	Wt																		
		Reps																		
Lunge	Quads/Hams/Calves	Wt																		
		Reps																		
Chest Press	Chest/Triceps	Wt																		
		Reps																		
Shoulder Press	Shoulders	Wt																		
		Reps																		
Butterfly	Lats/Traps	Wt																		
		Reps																		
Dumbbell Fly	Chest	Wt																		
		Reps																		
Biceps Curl	Biceps	Wt																		
		Reps																		
Triceps Ext.	Triceps	Wt																		
		Reps																		
		Wt																		
		Reps																		
		Wt																		
		Reps																		
		Wt																		
		Reps																		
		Wt																		
		Reps																		
		Wt																		
		Reps																		
		Wt																		
		Reps																		

Comments about these two weeks

_____

_____

_____

_____

Strength Training Log

Exercise	Target Area	Set	Week # 21 Day 1 1 2 3	Day 2 1 2 3	Day 3 1 2 3	Week # 22 Day 1 1 2 3	Day 2 1 2 3	Day 3 1 2 3
Squat	Quads/Hams/Gluts	Wt						
		Reps						
Lunge	Quads/Hams/Calves	Wt						
		Reps						
Chest Press	Chest/Triceps	Wt						
		Reps						
Shoulder Press	Shoulders	Wt						
		Reps						
Butterfly	Lats/Traps	Wt						
		Reps						
Dumbbell Fly	Chest	Wt						
		Reps						
Biceps Curl	Biceps	Wt						
		Reps						
Triceps Ext.	Triceps	Wt						
		Reps						
		Wt						
		Reps						
		Wt						
		Reps						
		Wt						
		Reps						
		Wt						
		Reps						
		Wt						
		Reps						
		Wt						
		Reps						

Comments about these two weeks

_____

_____

_____

_____

Strength Training Log

Exercise	Target Area	Set	Week # 23									Week # 24								
			Day 1			Day 2			Day 3			Day 1			Day 2			Day 3		
			1	2	3	1	2	3	1	2	3	1	2	3	1	2	3	1	2	3
Squat	Quads/Hams/Gluts	Wt																		
		Reps																		
Lunge	Quads/Hams/Calves	Wt																		
		Reps																		
Chest Press	Chest/Triceps	Wt																		
		Reps																		
Shoulder Press	Shoulders	Wt																		
		Reps																		
Butterfly	Lats/Traps	Wt																		
		Reps																		
Dumbbell Fly	Chest	Wt																		
		Reps																		
Biceps Curl	Biceps	Wt																		
		Reps																		
Triceps Ext.	Triceps	Wt																		
		Reps																		
		Wt																		
		Reps																		
		Wt																		
		Reps																		
		Wt																		
		Reps																		
		Wt																		
		Reps																		
		Wt																		
		Reps																		
		Wt																		
		Reps																		

Comments about these two weeks

"Limit 24-7" Guideline Log

	Limit Fat/"Bad" Carbs	2 Fruits	4 Vegetables	7 Grains (or less)	All 4? Yes/No
WEEK ONE					
Monday					
Tuesday					
Wednesday					
Thursday					
Friday					
Saturday					
Sunday					
Weekly Total					
Weekly Target					5

Comments about this week

_____

_____

_____

_____

"Limit 24-7" Guideline Log

	Limit Fat/"Bad" Carbs	2 Fruits	4 Vegetables	7 Grains (or less)	All 4? Yes/No
WEEK TWO					
Monday					
Tuesday					
Wednesday					
Thursday					
Friday					
Saturday					
Sunday					
Weekly Total					
Weekly Target					5

Comments about this week

_____

_____

_____

_____

"Limit 24-7" Guideline Log

	Limit Fat/"Bad" Carbs	2 Fruits	4 Vegetables	7 Grains (or less)	All 4? Yes/No
WEEK THREE					
Monday					
Tuesday					
Wednesday					
Thursday					
Friday					
Saturday					
Sunday					
Weekly Total					
Weekly Target					5

Comments about this week

_____

_____

_____

_____

"Limit 24-7" Guideline Log

	Limit Fat/"Bad" Carbs	2 Fruits	4 Vegetables	7 Grains (or less)	All 4? Yes/No
WEEK FOUR					
Monday					
Tuesday					
Wednesday					
Thursday					
Friday					
Saturday					
Sunday					
Weekly Total					
Weekly Target					5

Comments about this week

_____

_____

_____

_____

"Limit 24-7" Guideline Log

	Limit Fat/"Bad" Carbs	2 Fruits	4 Vegetables	7 Grains (or less)	All 4? Yes/No
WEEK FIVE					
Monday					
Tuesday					
Wednesday					
Thursday					
Friday					
Saturday					
Sunday					
Weekly Total					
Weekly Target					5

Comments about this week

_____

_____

_____

_____

"Limit 24-7" Guideline Log

	Limit Fat/"Bad" Carbs	2 Fruits	4 Vegetables	7 Grains (or less)	All 4? Yes/No
WEEK SIX					
Monday					
Tuesday					
Wednesday					
Thursday					
Friday					
Saturday					
Sunday					
Weekly Total					
Weekly Target					5

Comments about this week

_____

_____

_____

_____

"Limit 24-7" Guideline Log

	Limit Fat/"Bad" Carbs	2 Fruits	4 Vegetables	7 Grains (or less)	All 4? Yes/No
WEEK SEVEN					
Monday					
Tuesday					
Wednesday					
Thursday					
Friday					
Saturday					
Sunday					
Weekly Total					
Weekly Target					5

Comments about this week

_____

_____

_____

_____

"Limit 24-7" Guideline Log

	Limit Fat/"Bad" Carbs	2 Fruits	4 Vegetables	7 Grains (or less)	All 4? Yes/No
WEEK EIGHT					
Monday					
Tuesday					
Wednesday					
Thursday					
Friday					
Saturday					
Sunday					
Weekly Total					
Weekly Target					5

Comments about this week

_____

_____

_____

_____

"Limit 24-7" Guideline Log

	Limit Fat/"Bad" Carbs	2 Fruits	4 Vegetables	7 Grains (or less)	All 4? Yes/No
WEEK NIINE					
Monday					
Tuesday					
Wednesday					
Thursday					
Friday					
Saturday					
Sunday					
Weekly Total					
Weekly Target					5

Comments about this week

_____

_____

_____

_____

"Limit 24-7" Guideline Log

	Limit Fat/"Bad" Carbs	2 Fruits	4 Vegetables	7 Grains (or less)	All 4? Yes/No
WEEK TEN					
Monday					
Tuesday					
Wednesday					
Thursday					
Friday					
Saturday					
Sunday					
Weekly Total					
Weekly Target					5

Comments about this week

_____

_____

_____

_____

"Limit 24-7" Guideline Log

	Limit Fat/"Bad" Carbs	2 Fruits	4 Vegetables	7 Grains (or less)	All 4? Yes/No
WEEK ELEVEN					
Monday					
Tuesday					
Wednesday					
Thursday					
Friday					
Saturday					
Sunday					
Weekly Total					
Weekly Target					5

Comments about this week

"Limit 24-7" Guideline Log

	Limit Fat/"Bad" Carbs	2 Fruits	4 Vegetables	7 Grains (or less)	All 4? Yes/No
WEEK TWELVE					
Monday					
Tuesday					
Wednesday					
Thursday					
Friday					
Saturday					
Sunday					
Weekly Total					
Weekly Target					5

Comments about this week

_____

_____

_____

_____

INDEX

ABOUT THE AUTHOR

Bob Greene is an exercise physiologist and certified personal trainer specializing in fitness, metabolism, and weight loss. He has been a guest on *The Oprah Winfrey Show.* He is also a contributing writer and editor for *O The Oprah Magazine,* and writes on health and fitness for Oprah.com. Greene is the bestselling author of *Make the Connection, Get With the Program!, The Get With the Program! Daily Journal,* and *The Get With the Program! Guide to Good Eating.*

You can visit Bob Greene at his website, www.getwiththeprogram.org.